food
body &
love

"*Food, Body, & Love Companion Workbook* is a unique resource for people struggling with binge eating disorder and related problems, and for clinicians trying to help them break through these obsessive and self-defeating patterns of behavior. Anderson utilizes her experience and training as a body-based therapist, translating the principles and practices of Polyvagal Theory into a workbook that is user friendly and well-organized, with quotes, activities, illustrations, and group discussion topics enhancing the messages. The workbook teaches readers how to attain the tranquility and serenity known as the Ventral Vagal State and the essential elements of self-care. Using this Workbook may break down the shame that inevitably accompanies eating disorders while building self -compassion and new ways to manage lifelong negative habits surrounding food, eating and anxiety. There are a lot of golden nuggets in the workbook! Spoiler Alert: self-care requires more than a trip to the nail salon for a mani-pedi. Instead, pick up *Food, Body, & Love Companion Workbook* and you may find some true healing and hope for a life free of eating disorders."

Margo Maine, PhD, FAED, CEDS, has specialized in the treatment of eating disorders for 40 years. Author of *Hair Tells a Story: Hers, Yours, & Ours* (2023), and *Pursuing Perfection: Eating Disorders, Body Myths, and Women at Midlife and Beyond* (2016) and 6 other books related to eating disorders, she is a Founder and former Adviser of the National Eating Disorders Association and Founder and Fellow of the Academy for Eating Disorders, among other professional activities.

"Love. A must read for anyone – not just those struggling with eating disorders. *Food, Body & Love Companion Workbook* engages the reader with a combination of eight sessions offering stories, activities, journaling, reflections, values, habits and more. No stone is left unturned."

Adrienne Ressler, LMSW, CEDS, F.iaedp
Vice President, Professional Development, The Renfrew Center Foundation

"I loved it! Now, I want to read the *Food, Body & Love, but the greatest of these is love* book."

Vickie Berkus MD, eating disorder psychiatry.

"WELL-ORGANIZED, USER FRIENDLY, & COMPELLING – *Food, Body & Love Companion Workbook* illuminates with fresh insights linking neuroscience, mindfulness, nutrition, and self-care to create a solution to disordered eating. This illustrated workbook is a heartfelt and compassionate tool that will help many who struggle with food and body challenges through its delivery of an informed and inspired message."

Ralph E. Carson, RD, CEDS, PhD
Author of *The Brain Fix: What's the Matter with Your Grey Matter*
Senior Clinical and Research Advisor Eating Recovery Center/Pathlight

"Wow, Anderson's approach through this *Food, Body & Love Companion Workbook* is one that blends compassion and science yet feels simple and reachable. For the first time, the Polyvagal Theory is described in a way that feels accessible and solution focused. It's almost as if a beloved and trusted adult is guiding the scared parts to safety saying *"here, take my hand and we'll go on this journey TOGETHER. I'll show you some fun tricks that will help you find the calm you are seeking around food and eating."* As a professional working in private practice and with a pulse on modalities available for folks with food concerns, it was easy to envision clients responding to the simple explanations and finding healing in the practices and connections. I highly recommend this workbook to all who have been activated by the food insecurity that is baked into diet culture; there is hope and there is a way out!"

> Beth Harrell, MS, RDN, CEDS-S
> Host of The SeasonED RD Podcast for Professionals

"Food, Body & Love Companion Workbook is a creative, engaging and incredibly valuable tool for individuals struggling with body image and eating issues, as well as for those who want to build a better relationship with food, body, and self. Anderson, an experienced clinician, and leader in the field, draws on her own experience, in-depth knowledge and various modalities that truly work. This workbook is written in a compassionate and non-judgmental way that is easy to read, informative, and practical in its usefulness. Anderson nails it first by validating and making you feel understood and then provides prompts and exercises for self-reflection, a road map to understand your struggles and self, and then concrete solutions to support your journey. I look forward to both gifting this book and using it in my private practice with individuals and groups."

> Dena Cabrera, PsyD., CEDS-S
> Cabrera Psychological Services
> Past-President iaedp™

"Food, Body, & Love Companion Workbook deserves the lifetime achievement award for therapist authors. Each chapter, or Session, provides a thoughtful explanation of an aspect of healing our relationship with food and body, along with solutions to consider. Each page is a wealth of wisdom and guidance with easy-to-understand exercises and activities of self-care. Anyone who takes the time to go through this workbook step-by-step at their own pace will find healing by the time they reach the last page. It's a treasure trove....and Anderson's vulnerability in sharing her story in Food, Body & Love, but the greatest is love as a healing journey, and then offering it to the world is so beautiful."

Robyn Vogel, psychotherapist, founder of Come Back To Love®.

"Anderson has done it again, and this time it's a masterpiece. I have successfully worked with over one hundred clients and groups combined using Anderson's first book and workbook she coauthored with Michelle May, Eat What You Love, Love What You Eat for Binge Eating. Now, with Food Body & Love, but the greatest of these is love and its Companion Workbook she combines the science of eating disorders, neurobiology, best practice treatment modalities, compassion, and thoughtful, practical skills to help our clients find healing in their relationship with food and bodies. She takes great care to help the reader understand their behaviors through a lens of safety, love, and acceptance. Anderson continues to use her gifts to change lives. I highly recommend this Companion Workbook to anyone with a challenging relationship with food and their body."

Nancy Romanick RD, MBA, LPC
Nancy Romanick Counseling

"Food, Body & Love Companion Workbook by Anderson – provides practical solutions for self-discovery and healing your relationship with food and your body. You will learn to improve vagal tone through meditation, mindfulness, breathing, and other healing strategies. By combining science, wisdom, and a broad psychological knowledge base, this book offers step-by-step guidance to a healthier and happier you. I highly recommend this creative, practical, and user-friendly workbook."

> Delia Aldridge, MD, FAPA, CEDS-S
> Medical Director, Chicago Suburbs & Cincinnati Eating
> Recovery Center/ Pathlight
> Clinical Assistant Professor, Psychiatry & Behavioral Science Chicago
> Medical School, Rosalind Franklin University

"Having been in the world of sports medicine, I encounter disordered eating in my work with athletes on every level. I find Anderson's *Food, Body & Love Companion Workbook* very comprehensive and easy to read. In the realm of eating disorders, her approach is broken down into fundamentals in a tactful and empathic way. I highly recommend her literary work for anybody who is dealing with this disorder, or professionals managing this population. "

> David Carfagno DO CAQSM
> Scottsdale Sports Medicine Institute

"There are numerous gems in *Food, Body & Love Companion Workbook*, I have done many of the activities myself and share them in my work with clients. The sections I have found the most helpful include nervous system mapping (vagus nerve education) and evaluating the anatomy of a habit, as these concepts have offered invaluable discussion and reflection topics in my work with clients.

Anderson offers complex concepts in an easy to digest format, providing countless opportunities for the individual to reflect, process and heal."

>Megan A. Kniskern MS, RD, CEDS-S
>MAC Nutrition Services, Faculty Arizona State University

"Anderson's *Food Body & Love Companion Workbook* is an excellent workbook for the individual who struggles with their own relationship with food, body and accepting themselves. I love the solutions exercises that Anderson includes from meditation on all fronts, breath work, and becoming mindful when doing any of these healing activities. I can't wait to share this resource with clients as this workbook is a valuable resource in the field. Thank you for having a workbook to compliment your book, *Food, Body & Love, but the greatest of these is love!*"

>Robyn L. Goldberg, RDN, CEDS-S
>Author of *The Eating Disorder Trap* and Podcast

"I can't wait to use this *Food, Body & Love Companion Workbook* with my clients. As a Dietitian who has worked in the field of eating disorders for over three decades and has watched different treatment modalities come and go, I LOVE that this workbook weaves in science and its application as it pertains to the human experience of feeling dysregulated with food. I believe my clients will truly appreciate that this workbook compliments science-based nutrition with its therapeutic principles. As they work through chapter by chapter, they will experience validation in science and find support in the words that explain what they have been experiencing for so long, *finally*. This will be one of my top recommended workbooks."

>Kristine Sinner MS, RDN, LD/N, CEDS-S and Owner *Sinnergy Wellness Group*

"*Food, Body, & Love Companion Workbook* offers an integrative approach to addressing binge eating and other dysregulated relationships with food and one's body that assists the readers in exploring their experiences with more curiosity and compassion. Anderson incorporates elements from several theories in a relatable style, offers practical information, and provides tips to begin befriending your nervous system. Readers will appreciate the easily useable self-care solutions and activities to practice becoming more collaborative partners with their nervous systems and create more effective means of coping."

Michelle Gebhardt, Psy.D, CEDS-S
Clinical Director, Mindful Psychology Associates

"The *Food, Body, & Love Companion Workbook* will not only change the way you see yourself, but it will also positively shift the relationship you have with food and your body. Through activities, stories and thought provoking self-inquiring prompts the reader feels validated and understood, which provides them with a safe space to explore new ways of thinking, feeling, and behaving. I especially loved the self-care and mindfulness solution sections that provide tangible daily practices to help build new supportive habits. I am grateful to know this workbook is available, as it will help my clients on their journey to a life of peace with food, body freedom and self-love. "

Anne Poirier, Author of '*The Body Joyful*'
Director of Behavioral Health, Hilton Head Health

"If you've read Anderson's memoir, *Food, Body & Love, but the greatest of these is love*, this *Companion Workbook* will bring the concepts to life and help you begin to implement them in your own life, and it's a wonderful stand-alone resource too! If you are ready to examine, understand, and begin to change your relationship with food and body, the activities in this workbook are what you've been waiting for. It is chock full of new ideas you can add to your self-care toolbox. You will walk away with solutions to equip you to live in LOVE, not fear. I highly recommend it!"

Erin L. Todd, Blogger and Podcaster, *Intuitive Eating for Christian Women*

"Anderson is the real deal when it comes to resolving (healing) disordered eating. Her decades of clinical experience shine through inside every page of the *Food, Body, & Love Companion Workbook*. This is a powerful guide that'll give you a process you can follow to take consistent action towards a new reality where food and body image issues no longer control your life."

Jessica Flint, MS
Founder and CEO of *Recovery Warriors*

"Bravo to Anderson. The *Food, Body, & Love Companion Workbook*, is a much needed and easy to use resource for anyone, not just for those struggling with food issues. This workbook is broken down into 8 sessions. Each session starts with a brief introduction of that session topic, then provides several self-discovery pen and paper activities, and ends with a summary and actionable solutions that move the reader in the direction of "love." The reader might benefit from first reading Anderson's book *Food, Body, and Love, but the greatest is love*, but it is not a prerequisite to do so. This workbook stands alone. This book can be considered self-help or can be a companion workbook to use with a therapist or clinician. A must read."

Eileen Stellefson Myers, MPH, RDN, LDN, CEDRD-S, FAND

"I loved the *Food, Body & Love Companion Workbook*! The exercises in it are very applicable to many of my clients and have been a great discussion starter in therapy. I also liked the way the tips are laid out in easy-to-follow steps. There are a lot of creative ways to cover the content of the book. "

Chandra Baylor, MS, LMFT, R-DMT, CEDS
Resilient Self Holistic Therapy Services

"*Food, Body & Love Companion Workbook* opened my eyes, heart, and body to an appreciation for myself. Finally, a REAL TOOL, not just a philosophy, to put into practice.   I feel seen and "normal" in my relationship with food for the first time. Don't rush into and through each exercise. Sit with it, go deep with it, let yourself be seen by yourself! You will not regret the journey. I am still 'doing the work' but see significant shifts in my patterns. While nutrition is science, it doesn't consider the individual mind which is much more powerful. Anderson blends science in understanding your impulses, cravings, and patterns with practical lessons in eating to unravel all the programming (conditioning) that is blurring your view of self."

Amy Flores-Young, Lifelong Learner
Disability Advocate, Concierge and Retreat Travel Professional

"Anderson has designed a practical evidence-based workbook relating mind, body, soul, and heart interconnection to your recovery from disordered eating. The *Food, Body & Love Companion Workbook* takes you through a clear understanding of the physiological reasons why you have food cravings to practical skills that help you implement new ways of calming. Integrating the Polyvagal Theory, the workbook offers ways to self-soothe, find balance, peace, and love for self, body, and food. The design works for individuals or groups in such a way that there is introspective journaling, skill application, and the ability for discussion promoting connection in each of the 8 sessions. It is an excellent and hands-on resource that I highly recommend. It is a companion to Anderson's powerful book, *"Food, Body & love, but the greatest of these is love."*

Amy E. Wasserbauer, Ph.D. CEDS-S
Assistant Director, Arizona State University Counseling Services

food
body &
love

companion workbook

Dr. Kari Anderson

In view of the complex, individual nature of health and fitness issues, this and the ideas, programs, processes, and suggestions are not intended to replace the advice of trained medical and behavioral health professionals. All matters regarding one's physical and mental health require medical supervision.

The authors' role is strictly educational in the context of this book and program materials. The author is not providing any assessments, individualized therapeutic interventions, or personal medical advice. Seek medical advice from your personal health care provider regarding your personal risks and benefits insofar as adopting the suggestions of this program.

Please consult with a trained eating disorder therapist if you have or think you have binge eating disorder, bulimia, or anorexia before engaging in this program. The author disclaims any liability arising directly or indirectly from the use of this book or program.

ISBN: 978-1-7377204-3-0

Published by Dr. Kari Anderson
Scottsdale, Arizona

Printer: Author2Market.com
Cover design: Keenly Interactive
Cover production: ElectronicInkAZ.com
Graphic Art and Layout: ElectronicInkAZ.com
Content Editing: Alisa Cooper Wechsler
Proofreading: Ann Narcisian Videan

dedication

I dedicate this workbook to anyone looking for safety. Once safe, may you find your authentic self, the one hidden behind food and other strongholds of protection.

contents

Solutions

Mindful Solutions

Meditations

Self-Care Solutions

Introduction

In 2021, I released my memoir; **Food, Body, & Love**, *but the greatest of these is love*. With a heavy dose of compassion combined with scientific theory, I explain my experience with binge eating from the viewpoint of my body rather than my emotions. Many felt understood for the first time, and their shame melted away as they resonated with my story. They were hungry for more, wanting practical details and simple steps for integrating healing into their own lives.

In 2022, I created a self-paced online course, *Food, Body and Love: A Compassionate and Science-Based Solution for Binge Eating*. I began leading groups and augmenting individual therapy with the strategies I detailed in my book. This *companion workbook* provides help and hope to those still struggling to find safety in their bodies. It's a user's guide for breaking free of the burden of obsessional cravings, impulsivity, and feelings of loss of control around food. I hope it finds you.

After working as an eating disorder specialist since the early 90s, I have seen many treatment trends over the years. I have had extensive training in mindfulness-based cognitive behavioral therapies such as DBT and ACT, and you will see evidence of these in many of the "Mindful Solutions" offered in this workbook.

I highlight the importance of mindfulness in the workbook because it is the most effective, evidence-based treatment for anxiety. Why focus on treatment for anxiety? Many believe, as I do, that eating disorders *are* anxiety disorders.

With ongoing training and studying, I have evolved into a body-based therapist. I wanted to delve deeper to discover the root cause of symptoms instead of just treating them. As a student, follower, and practitioner of Polyvagal Theory, I understand how our autonomic nervous system states influence our daily experiences. They influence our eating behaviors, social behaviors, learning behaviors...our world view.

I look at all symptomatic behaviors through the lens of safety verses fear. Finding safety is the key to resolving unwanted behaviors. Once we understand that our behaviors serve to protect us, we can approach ourselves with compassion.

This is an eclectic workbook using many different therapeutic modalities I have found effective with disordered eating. Many of the activities have been adapted from the work of others, and I gratefully acknowledge their contributions.

Although my personal experience was with Binge Eating Disorder, it is not necessary to have an eating disorder to benefit from this workbook. Over the years. I have heard the same experience described in different ways: "Feeling out of control with food, relentless food obsessions, sugar addiction, compulsive eating, chronic yo-yo dieting, stress or emotional eating..." It does not matter what you call it or how it manifests. What matters is you feel understood and can find relief.

If you have been diagnosed with an eating disorder or think you have an eating disorder, please reach out to an eating disorder specialist for help. You may use this workbook with the help of a trained professional.

How to Use this Workbook

The workbook consists of eight "Sessions." Each session contains a lesson, opportunity for reflective journaling, several activities, and a host of self-care solutions.

The "Solutions" pages are easily found as they have a grey mark on the outermost edge. These are visible on the unbound edge when the workbook is closed. Return to these pages often. They contain actionable solutions aimed at moving us away from our fear states and toward a state of love. You will learn how to harness and maintain your autonomic nervous system in a calm state of safety, love, and connection called *the ventral vagal state.*

This workbook highlights the 8 C's Experience: eight powerful words, all beginning with the letter C: Confident, Curious, Connected, Courageous, Compassionate, Clear, Creative, and Calm. These words remind us of the beautiful parts we can access when we are in the ventral vagal state. It is here you will find your most authentic self.

While the workbook does not follow the order of *Food, Body, & Love, but the greatest of these is love*, I do reference it when there is an opportunity to read more about a topic. Just look for the little circle stamp at the top of the lesson being presented. It will direct you where to go in the book. The workbook can be used and understood on its own, but your experience is enhanced by using the workbook as a "companion" to the book.

Lastly, at the end of each session, there are suggested questions for therapists and group leaders who want to use this workbook to facilitate a group. The group experience is invaluable because connection is key to healing the nervous system. This workbook is designed as a self-help tool, yet many professionals I have trained and supervised use these concepts in working with clients. I hope this workbook helps you find your authentic self, the one hidden behind food and other strongholds of protection.

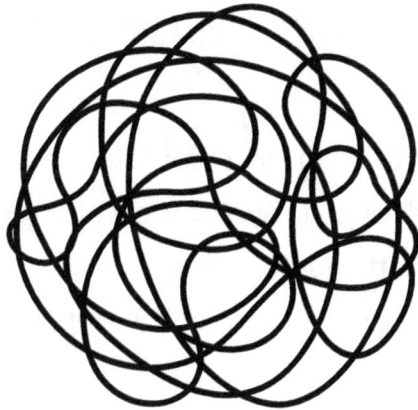

session one

"The irony is that we attempt to disown our difficult stories. To appear more whole or more acceptable, but our wholeness, even our wholeheartedness, actually depends on the integration of all our experiences, including our falls"

Brené Brown
Rising Strong

One Hot Mess

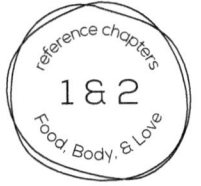

Everyone has a shameful story; I had many related to my behavior with food. I found once I began to speak about my stories, I started to shed the shame. When I stood back and observed it through a lens of science and compassion, I realized there were perfectly good explanations for my behavior.

Story Sharing

Share a story related to your behavior with food. Describe it as if you are past the shame and retelling the story from a place of understanding and compassion.

_____

_____

_____

_____

_____

_____

_____

_____

In the beginning... When I was eight years old, I began to sneak food (primarily sugar) and hide in isolation to eat it. It made me feel better.

I developed a pattern of turning to food to soothe myself. After all, we all just want to feel better and safer. Share a story about an early memory related to your pattern of turning to food to feel better.

You Mean There is a Name for This?

Binge Eating Disorder is the most common eating disorder, but it often goes unrecognized, underdiagnosed, and undertreated. Binge Eating Disorder has the following recurrent components. Check the ones that ring true for you:

- ☐ Eating large quantities of food, more than is considered normal for a specific time or situation.

- ☐ A feeling of losing control once you begin eating - especially certain foods.

- ☐ A feeling of self-loathing and disgust after a binge episode.

- ☐ Eating when not hungry or when already uncomfortably full.

- ☐ Eating alone due to shame about what and how much you are eating.

- ☐ Sometimes eating rapidly or feeling detached from the eating experience.

Comments

_____

_____

_____

_____

_____

Food Behavior Timeline

Activity

Disordered eating presents on a continuum of behavior. It tends to get progressively worse over time as you establish a stronger habit of eating for emotional relief.

Binge eating often starts as comfort eating, stress eating, and/or mindless eating. It can turn into loss-of-control-eating, and, for some, into food compulsion and a behavioral addiction. Binge eating has a strong restrictive component due to the pervasive drive for thinness, so some people have periods of restrictive dieting in their timeline.

Reflect on your historical journey with food and body. Create a timeline on the next page. List your age, any significant events at that time in your life, the eating behavior corresponding to that time, and body fluctuations, if applicable.

example

Age Span/Event

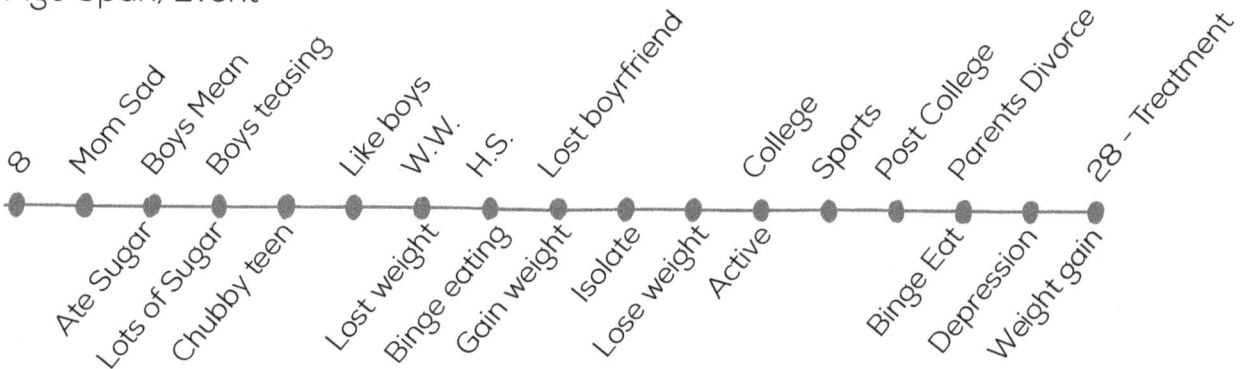

Above the line (left to right): 8, Mom Sad, Boys Mean, Boys teasing, Like boys, W.W., H.S., Lost boyfriend, College, Sports, Post College, Parents Divorce, 28 - Treatment

Below the line (left to right): Ate Sugar, Lots of Sugar, Chubby teen, Lost weight, Binge eating, Gain weight, Isolate, Lose weight, Active, Binge Eat, Depression, Weight gain

Behavior and Body Changes if any.

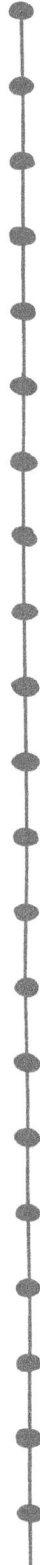

(Turn workbook sideways for more room)

Assessing Your Food and Body Relationships

Activity

Food Freedom vs. Body Care

In the diagram on the next page, we will explore two vectors that intersect to help assess your relationship with food and your body.

The vertical line indicates your relationship with food on a continuum from FREEDOM at the top to CONTROL on the bottom. Ask yourself, are you restrictive, rule-driven, and controlled in what you eat? If so, this indicates tight CONTROL. Or, do you allow food of any kind at any time you want it, without boundaries? This indicates the extreme of FOOD FREEDOM. Of course, your relationship with food can fall anywhere in between. While we all go to extremes sometimes, for this activity, assess your relationship with food based on what you do MOST of the time. Mark an X on the vertical line that best represents your current relationship with food.

Now, look at the horizontal line indicating your relationship with your body. The far left indicates NEGLECT of your physical body. Are you angry, disconnected, or even abusive toward yourself at times? The far right indicates impeccable CARE of your body. Do you listen, respond, and lean in with curiosity? Are you compassionate and have an attitude of respect for your body? Mark an X on the horizontal line best representing your current relationship with your body on the continuum. Draw a line connecting the two X's. This will identify which quadrant you typically fall into relating to your current relationship with food and your body.

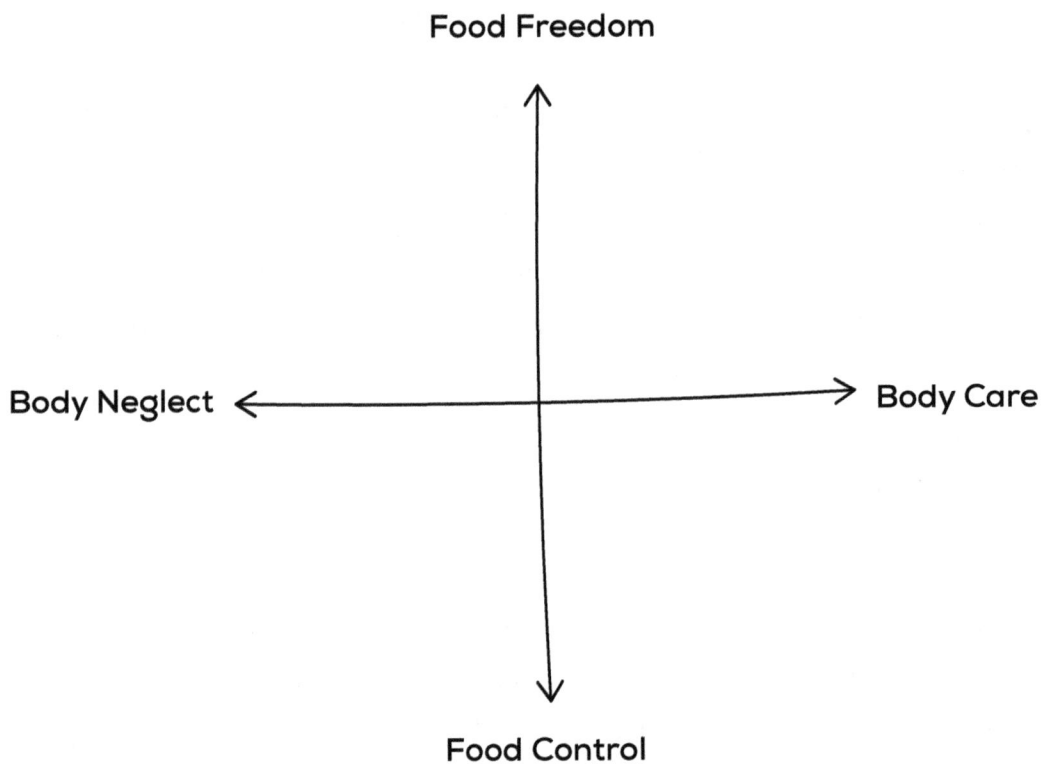

Food Freedom

Fear - Based
"Out of control"

Safety
"Freedom
and care"

Body Neglect ←   → **Body Care**

Fear - Based
"Abuse"

Fear - Based
"Trapped"

Food Control

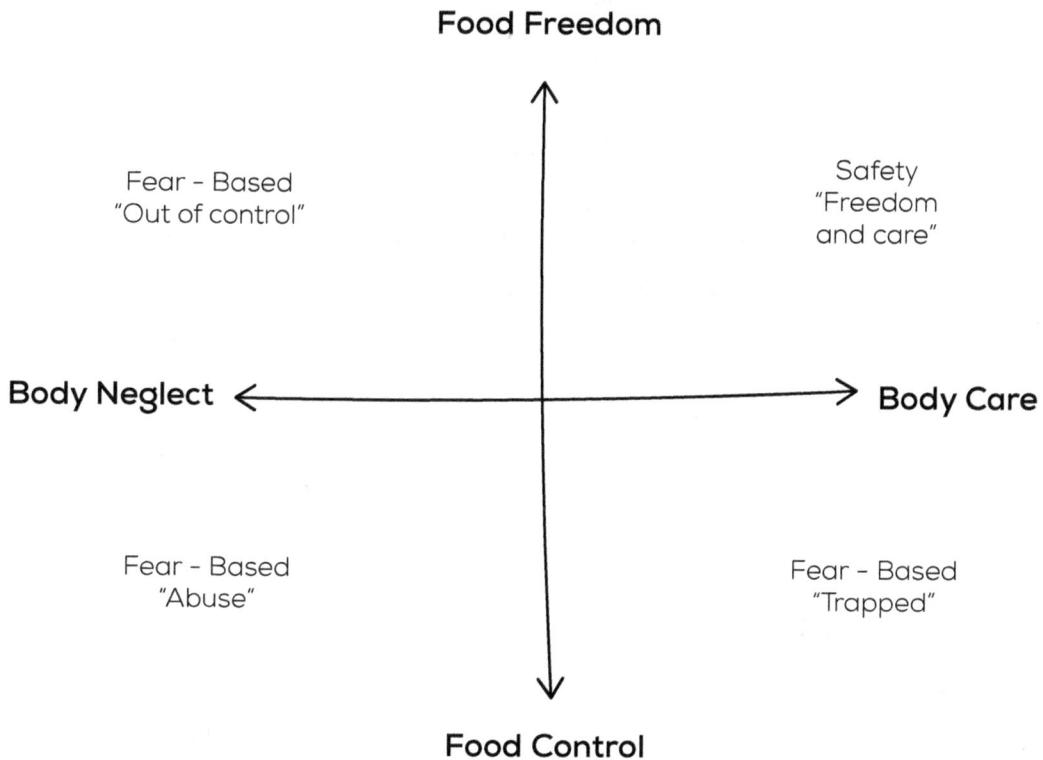

Adapted from Am I hungry?, P.L.L.C.

The top right-hand corner is a quadrant of safety. It reflects a balance of Freedom and Care, where flexible boundaries regarding food co-exist with consistent, loving self-care. It is the sweet spot we are working toward in this workbook.

The other three quadrants are fear-based. Those who land in the top left-hand corner tend to feel out of control, perhaps with an "I don't care" attitude. They usually respond with avoidance behavior or an urgent need to control. This is typically reflective of someone in a binge eating cycle.

The bottom left corner feels abusive, depicting behaviors seen in severe eating disorders like anorexia or bulimia. The bottom right-hand quadrant gives an illusion of control, but it tends to be driven by fear and anxiety. These people often feeling trapped, a typical scenario for those with orthorexia.

Mindful Solutions

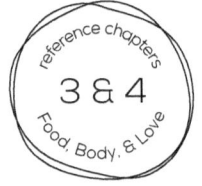

solution

Mindfulness

Mindfulness provides us with a heightened ability to simply observe feelings and experiences, take charge of decisions and disengage automatic reactivity. It's accepting whatever happens because you can't control anything but your own self and, in turn, living intentionally with purpose.

It is simply present-moment awareness without judgment.

Mindfulness bridges the gap from extrinsic to intrinsic motivation, which is necessary to listen to our body's wisdom and the values of our heart, steering away from the extrinsic rules and cultural judgments that create fear, comparison, and doubt in us. Mindfulness involves experimentation with curiosity, observation of feedback loops, and choosing a valued direction or path. Mindfulness is a journey. Won't you come with me?

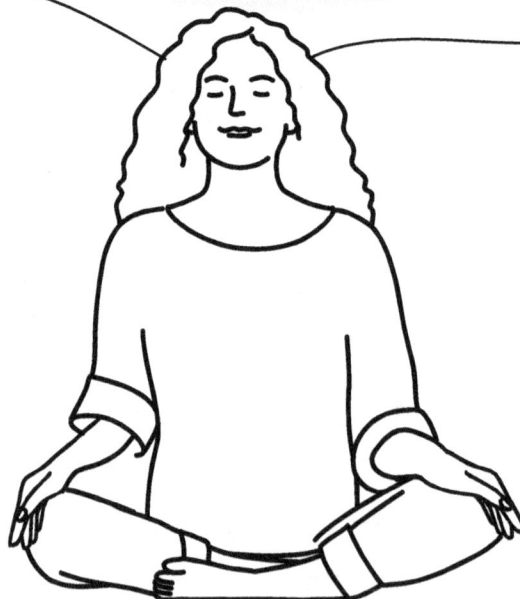

Mindful Solutions

"True self-care is not bubble baths and bon bons. It is making the choice to build a life you don't need to regularly escape from."

Brianna Wiest

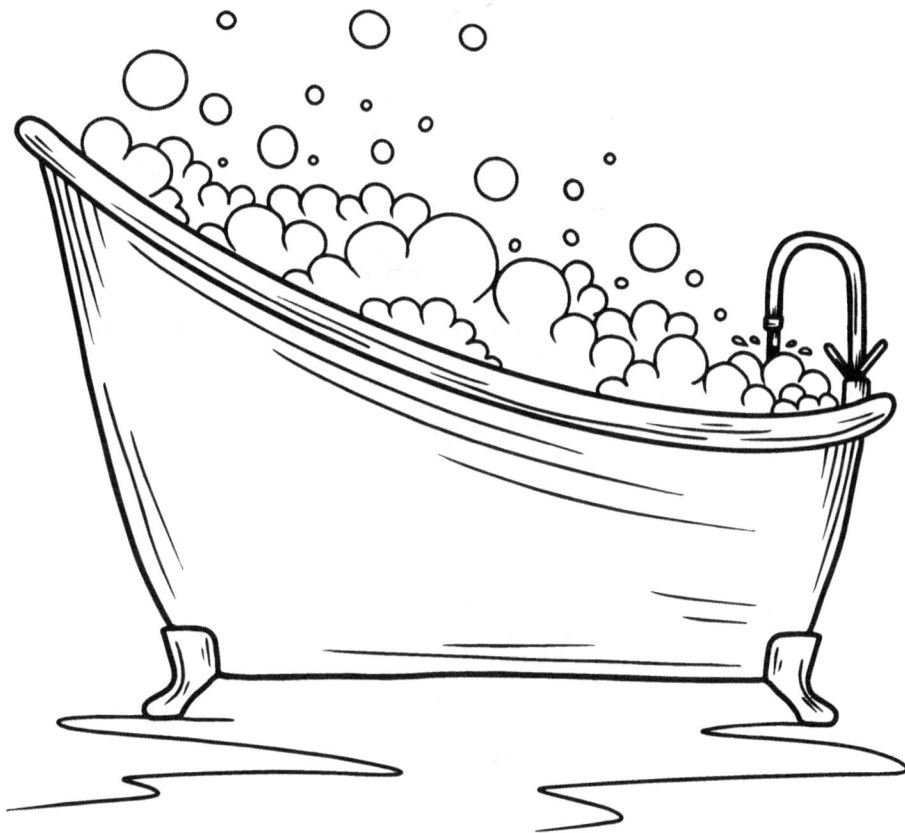

Experiential Avoidance vs. Acceptance

Experiential Avoidance

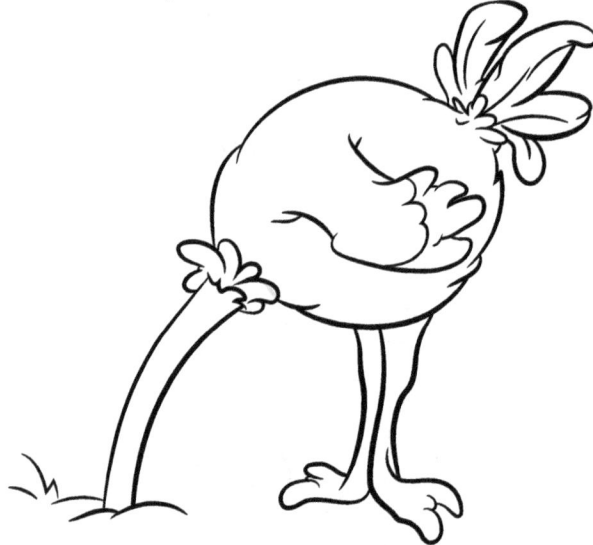

An attempt or desire to suppress unwanted internal experiences, such as emotions, thoughts, memories, and bodily experiences.

Acceptance

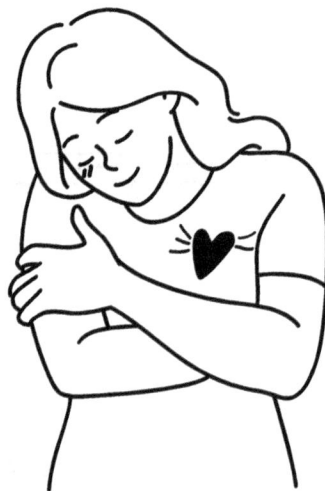

Allowing your internal experiences to occur without trying to change them or ignore them.

Journal

1. How have you used food to escape or avoid discomfort?

_____

_____

_____

_____

_____

_____

2. What strategies could you use to help end the struggle with acceptance?

_____

_____

_____

_____

_____

_____

solution

3. List the things you could learn to accept, understanding they are not directly under your control.

_____

_____

_____

_____

_____

_____

_____

4. What can you change that is within your control?

_____

_____

_____

_____

_____

_____

Self-Care Solutions

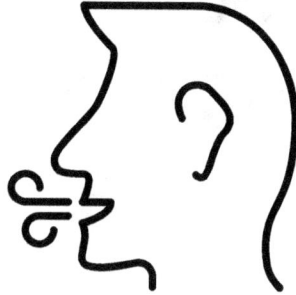

Breathe

Exhale

Notice spontaneous sighs

Use intentional sighs

Blow up an imaginary balloon or blow out imaginary candles

Slow abdominal breathing decreases heart rate

Sing!

Play a wind instrument

Laugh!

solution

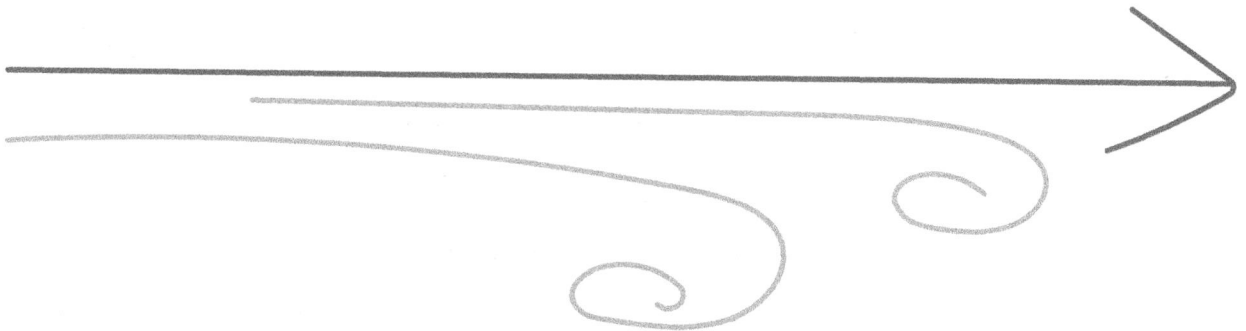

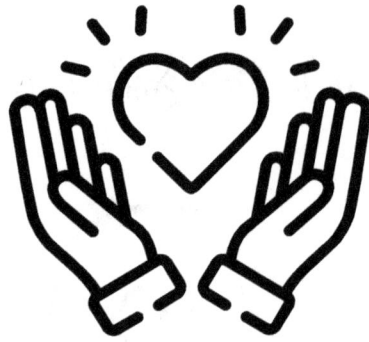

Gratitude

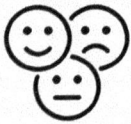

It can co-exist with other feelings. We can feel disappointed and grateful. One does not exclude the other.

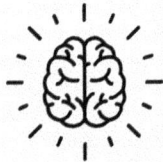

It changes our brain structure. We feel more peace and less reactive and defensive.

Keep a gratitude journal, list, or a photo journal.

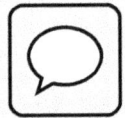

Send thank you notes or a "thinking of you" text.

Create a gratitude journal. List people and things you are grateful for. Think and daydream about these things. Revisit often and add to the list.

_____

_____

_____

_____

_____

_____

Gratitude Journal

_____

_____

_____

_____

_____

_____

_____

_____

_____

_____

_____

_____

_____

_____

_____

_____

_____

_____

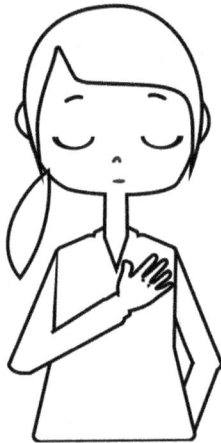

Combining Breathing and Gratitude

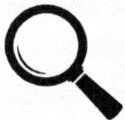

Focus your attention on the area of your heart.

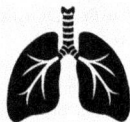

Begin to breathe slowly and deeply in a smooth easy rhythm, as if you are breathing through the heart.

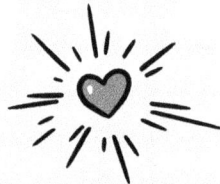

At the same time, begin to capture a genuine feeling of love, care, and appreciation, as if it is radiating from your heart.

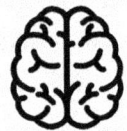

This technique aligns your heart rhythms into a more coherent pattern, creating a state of clarity and connection.

Adapted from Quick Coherence Technique, Heartmath

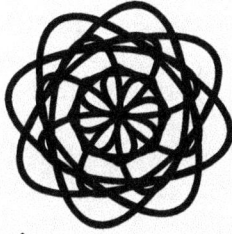

8 C's

Experience

In this session we will focus on Courage.

"Be Courageous"

Draw a picture or symbol, or write a phrase, reminding and anchoring you to the feeling of courage.

Reflect and list the courageous acts you have carried out in the past. What would you do if you weren't afraid?

_____

_____

_____

How can you create more safety in your life so you can be more courageous?

_____

_____

_____

Reflection and Discussion

Reflection: Space for free writing on this chapter's insights.

_____

_____

_____

_____

_____

_____

_____

_____

_____

_____

_____

_____

_____

_____

_____

_____

_____

_____

Discussion and Activities for Group Leaders

- Ask if anyone, or all, would care to share a story or their history timeline. Tend to feelings.

- Ask group members to share their relationship graph and what they learned from doing the activity. What would it be like to live in the Freedom and Care quadrant? What possibilities might open up?

- Discuss avoidance vs. acceptance behavior. Have each person mention an avoidance behavior and how it could be turned into an acceptance behavior. For example: I walked into the room and did not make eye contact with anyone. I could have walked in and looked around with a smile on my face.

- Implement some of the "Self-Care Solutions." Practice abdominal breathing and breathing from the heart. Sing a verse or two from a song everyone knows. For example: "Michael Row the Boat Ashore," "You're a Grand Old Flag," etc. Have the group exaggerate pretend laughter until everyone is actually laughing.

- Gratitude Activity: Have the group stand in a circle. Throw a beanbag to someone. When they catch it, they have to say something they are grateful for. Then they toss the beanbag to someone else until everyone has had a chance to share.

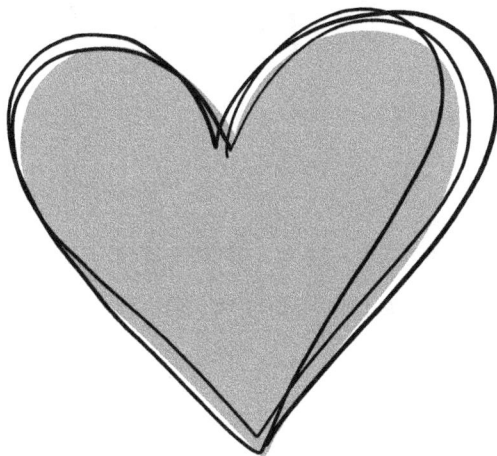

session two

" The more I learn about science, the
more I believe in God."

Albert Einstein

The Love Code

STRESS, THE BODY AND YOUR
EATING BEHAVIOR

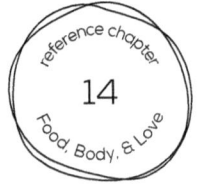

"I've never met anyone who doesn't have a good reason for their disordered eating behaviors." Science validates the reality of your struggle. When you understand the nervous system and how it works, you gain an appreciation for your struggle with food. When we experience the sensation of fear in our bodies, it's uncomfortable. Everything in our being tries to find safety. Biologically, eating provides a natural calming sensation. It allows the body to shift into a "rest and digest" nervous system state, neurologically mimicking the feeling of being in relationship and connected to others. It calms the fear of being alone.

Our bodies were designed to co-exist and co-regulate with others, so being alone is a threat to our survival. Many people don't feel safe, and food can become a place of safety for them. If stress-eating increases the size of your body, often a protective response, the culture we live in passes judgment on us and drives us further into isolation.

Our nervous system has a built-in, subconscious system for detecting safety and danger. Some people's nervous systems are more tuned into danger because of their family history or their own traumatic experiences. Their systems are wired for protection rather than for connection. The world is scary to them, and they tend to experience physically noticeable fear states throughout the day and night. They may be labeled as "sensitive" or diagnosed with anxiety or depression, but their body is just defending itself from the experience of fear. Your behaviors only represent your efforts to feel better and safer.

How does feeling fearful and apprehensive influence your own eating behavior? Does writing about it change the way you feel about it, or about yourself?

_____

_____

_____

_____

_____

_____

_____

_____

_____

_____

_____

_____

_____

_____

_____

_____

_____

_____

The Vagus Nerve

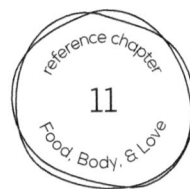

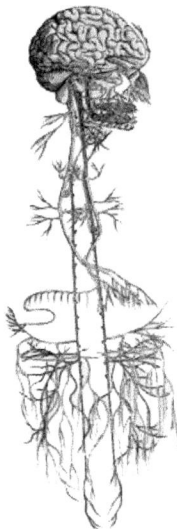

The vagus nerve is the master regulator of the body. It is the tenth of twelve cranial nerves that make up our social engagement system, and the most famous by far. It is the longest nerve in the body with branches going to the muscles of the face, throat, heart, lungs, and the digestive system.

With its complex web of nerves in our belly, the vagus serves as the communication highway between the gut and the brain. When it is functioning well, it "puts the brakes on" our physical fear responses so we can experience safety and connection to access the best parts of ourselves. Keep in mind, we operate best in a state of love.

When we feel safe and connected, the body doesn't have to use its energy to stay hypervigilant and defensive. When our vagal nerve is healthy—has "vagal tone"—we are open to an entire world of possibilities. When the vagus nerve is not functioning well, or we have poor vagal tone, the body exists in a fear state where health issues, both mental and physical, develop over time. In this session, we will explore, map, and begin to shift our fear states into states of safety.

Things That Go Bump in the Night

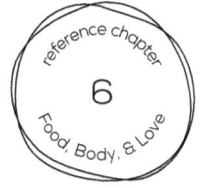

reference chapter

6

Food, Body, & Love

Neuroscientists have studied the effects of childhood trauma, real or perceived, on the nervous system. Adverse Childhood Events (ACEs) make us more vulnerable and sensitive to the effects of stress on the nervous system, and, ultimately, on our health. Our nervous system can also be compromised by events occurring in adulthood. All traumatic events can bring on symptoms of stress and anxiety, or a diagnosis of Post-Traumatic Stress Disorder (PTSD). If you have experienced trauma or adverse events of any kind, you might want to consider working with a trauma-informed therapist.

In my book, I discuss my early infancy/childhood experiences and grade school sexual boundary violations that interfered with my sense of safety, trust, and my beliefs regarding men, women, and power. I'm not asking you to do a deep dive here, but if you feel safe enough, reflect on some adverse events in your life which may have "imprinted" fear and apprehension into your nervous system.

_____

_____

_____

_____

_____

_____

_____

_____

_____

Mapping Your Nervous System

Activity

Our autonomic nervous system is divided into two branches: Sympathetic and Parasympathetic. According to Polyvagal Theory, there is a third branch, the vagal branch, controlled by the vagus nerve. The vagal branch has ventral and dorsal aspects, giving rise to the name "polyvagal" for its multiple components. Whew, anatomy out of the way!

A polyvagal-informed trauma therapist, Deb Dana, LCSW, connects the anatomy to human function by using a ladder. The ladder represents where you are in regard to which part of your autonomic nervous system is activated at the time. The diagram below is an adaptation of that concept.

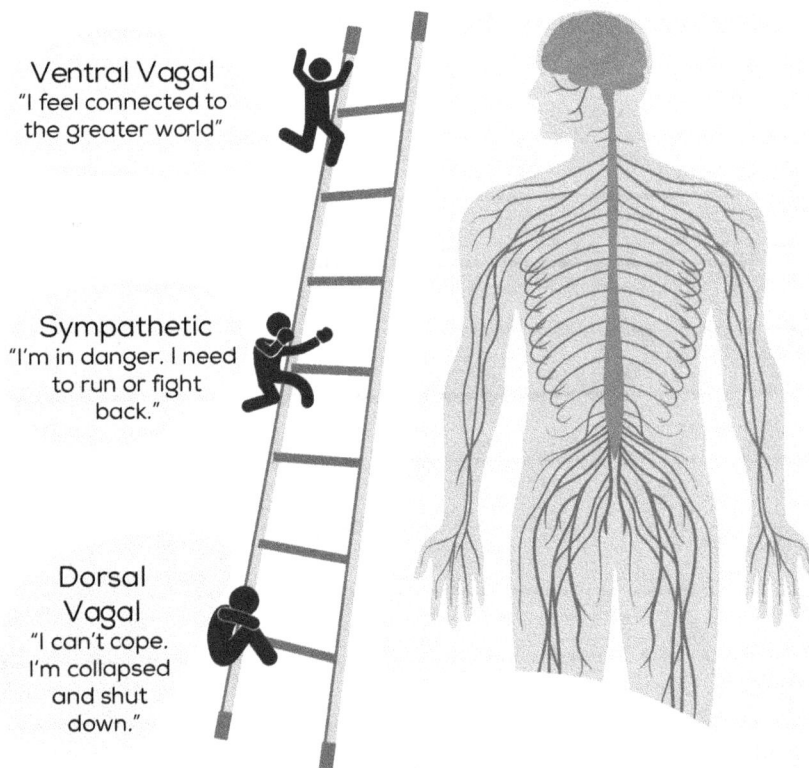

Ventral Vagal
"I feel connected to the greater world"

Sympathetic
"I'm in danger. I need to run or fight back."

Dorsal Vagal
"I can't cope. I'm collapsed and shut down."

Mapping Your Nervous System:
Creating language for your body's experience.

The following three pathways offer some language to get you started thinking about these autonomic states.

VENTRAL VAGAL

All my best parts are available to me.

- Confident
- Curious
- Connected
- Courageous
- Compassionate
- Clear
- Creative
- Calm

I'm in a place of love, joy, and hope that's filled with energy.

SYMPATHETIC

I'm distracted. I can't think. I feel uneasy.

- Edgy
- Tense
- Worried
- Chaotic
- Overwhelmed
- Panicked
- Annoyed
- Frustrated
- Jealous
- Disgusted
- Furious
- Enraged

I can't breathe.

DORSAL VAGAL

I've escaped and collapsed into a place of:

- Shame
- Emptiness
- Hopelessness
- Despair
- Numbness

I feel:
- Stuck
- Shut down
- Frozen
- Dissociated
- Exhausted

Everything is hard.

Describe what it feels like when you are at the top of the ladder. Can you remember a time when you felt that way? If not, can you imagine what it might feel like to be at the top of the ladder? Describe it in detail.

_____

_____

_____

_____

_____

Describe what it feels like when you are falling down the ladder. When is the last time you felt like that? Describe it in detail.

_____

_____

_____

_____

_____

_____

Describe what it feels like when you are at the bottom of the ladder. Can you remember the last time you were there? Describe it in detail.

_____

_____

_____

_____

_____

_____

Mapping Your Nervous System:
Creating your own "PET scan" of your nervous system.

Begin by spending some time in a relaxed and meditative state. Then reflect on recent memories of each of the three autonomic states. Use crayons or colored pencils to depict what your body feels like in these distinct autonomic pathways. Think of each experience as energy moving and changing within the body. Use darker or lighter shades depending on the intensity and location of this energy in your body. Create your own colorful map, or pet scan, to represent the experience you had. Give each picture a caption or a name to label the experience.

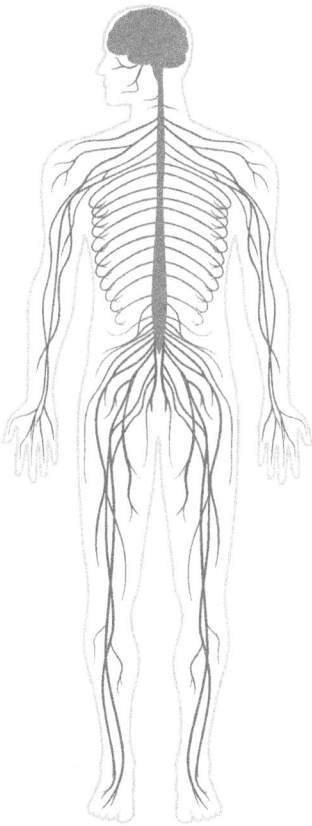 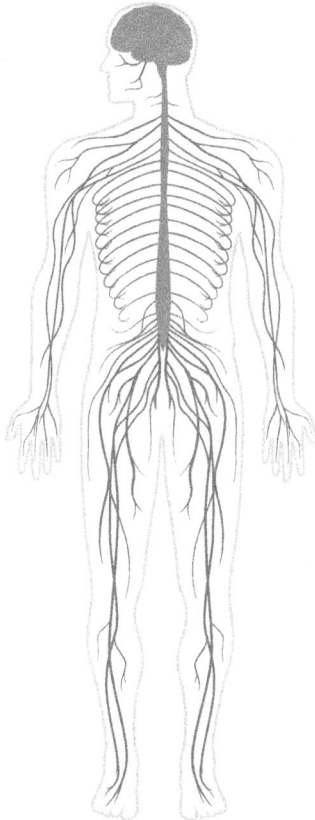 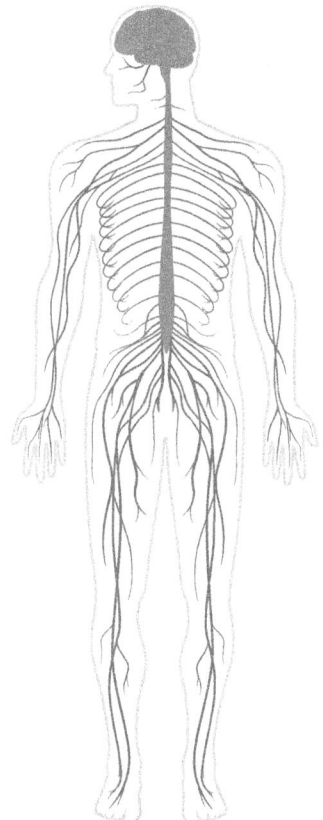

Ventral Vagal   Sympathetic   Dorsal Vagal

Befriending Your Nervous System

Activity

As you continue with your mindful exploration of your body's internal experience, I encourage you to be curious and less fearful of these states of energy. As you embrace these body scans rather than pull away from them, you will notice the energy breaks up and flows more readily.

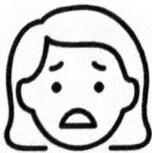

Your nervous system responds to fear. It is protective. Befriend it, meaning embrace the energy with curiosity and compassion.

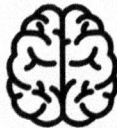

Attend to your autonomic nervous system (ANS) by identifying its states. Name them and recognize how your body moves in and out of these different states.

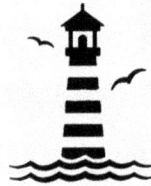

Track your states throughout the day. Notice how triggers and twinkle lights influence each state.

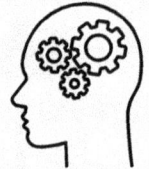

Influence your ANS with intentional practices.

Your nervous system is designed to respond to fear. It is protective. Embracing all nervous system states with curiosity and compassion, even those reacting to fear, is called *befriending*. "Thank you for giving me the heads up something might be wrong."

Track your states throughout the day. Stay curious about which experiences, or actions influence each nervous system state. Notice how things that trigger fearful responses influence your states versus the effect of *twinkle light experiences.

*More on twinkle lights later in "Self-Care Solutions."

Attend to your autonomic nervous system (ANS) by identifying its three states. Name them and recognize how your body moves in and out of these states.

Influence your ANS with intentional practices—"Self-Care Solutions." These practices are empowering. They help you discover you are not a victim of your nervous system but rather a collaborative partner.

Ventral Vagal (Calm, connected)

How do I climb up here?

What self-care practices sustain my ability to maintain this position on the ladder?

_____

_____

_____

_____

_____

_____

_____

_____

_____

_____

_____

_____

_____

_____

Sympathetic ("Fight or Flight")

Which triggers make me slip down the rungs of the ladder?

What part of the day or night do I most often find myself here?

What do I notice about my body and emotions at that time?

What do I need when this happens?

What can I do to climb back up the ladder?

Dorsal Vagal (Collapsed, shut down, withdrawn)

What is happening when I fall down the ladder and can't get up?

What behaviors, thoughts, or circumstances contribute to this?

What can I do to move back up the ladder?

Hint: How do you mobilize when feeling stuck or frozen?

What can I do to prevent myself from falling to the bottom of the ladder?

_____

_____

_____

_____

_____

_____

_____

_____

_____

_____

_____

_____

_____

Self-Care Solutions

Twinkle Lights

Twinkle lights are things that can calm our sympathetic nervous system when it is activated and bring energy to the nervous system when it has collapsed into the dorsal vagal state. Twinkle lights serve as autonomic nervous system regulators. When we experience twinkle lights, we must breathe in and capture these micro-moments of "awe" within our nervous system's "memory." Many find twinkle lights in the beauty of nature or in the safe comforting face of a loved one.

Sensory Resourcing

Sensory input from our cranial nerves has a great influence on our autonomic state. For instance, cold temperatures can calm us down. Music can bring us to tears, and the sight of a sunrise or sunset can ground us to the rhythms of the universe. It is important to have an accessible tool kit full of sensory resources. Even micro-dosing throughout the day helps keep our autonomic nervous system regulated. Gazing out the window at a flower or a hummingbird, or seeing a gorgeous sunset can serve as micro doses of positive sensory input. Other sensory experiences can be planned, for instance macro dosing on nature over a weekend or weeklong vacation.

My Favorite Things

Brainstorm a list of all your favorite sensory experiences. Keep adding to the list as you go through this workbook. Return to these sensory experiences in your mind to help regulate your autonomic nervous system. Categorize each as a single sense (i.e. What do you like to see? What are the things you like to hear?), keeping in mind most experiences are multisensory. For instance, taste, smell, and texture all combine to create our eating experience. For the category of taste sensation, focus on flavors that either calm or energize you. Try to stay away from triggering foods.

See   *Hear*   *Feel*   *Smell*   *Taste*

Circle those things you can do daily.

Mindful Solutions

Self-Observing vs. Self-Narrative

Do you ever get caught up in your negative thoughts? We all do. Think of your thoughts as a self-narrative: the story your brain creates to help make sense of what you experience. Your narrative is based on the "software" that has been programmed into your mind. So, it is not necessarily true, real, or relevant to your life today. To free yourself of these thoughts, you must become an objective observer of them.

Mindfulness suggests you step away and notice what you are thinking. Try to shift into the role of nonjudgmental observer. Hmm... interesting. This is a bit abstract at first but, with practice, you can distance yourself from negative thinking and outdated belief systems. You can simply observe your thoughts. You can even choose what you want to think. How liberating is that? Ariana Grande sings, "Thank you, next!"

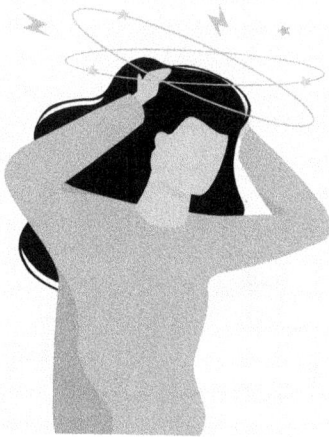

Self-Narrative
I am what I think.

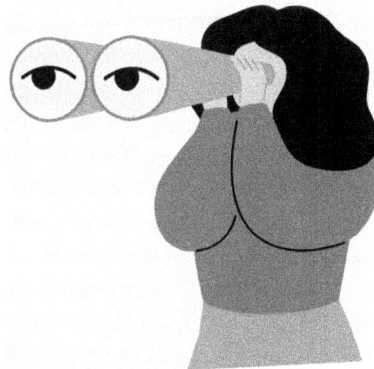

Self-Observing
I'm noticing what I'm thinking.

Mindful Solutions

Body Scan Meditation

The body scan meditation is a method of moving inside and observing our physical and emotional experiences and responses. The ability to do so is called interoception. So, interoception allows us to notice the signals our body gives us about how it feels and what it needs. It can tell us, through the energy of fear, if something isn't quite right. It signals whether we are hungry or full, or sick. It tells us whether we are tired, sad, content, or happy. We just have to slow down, listen, and pay attention. Here's how:

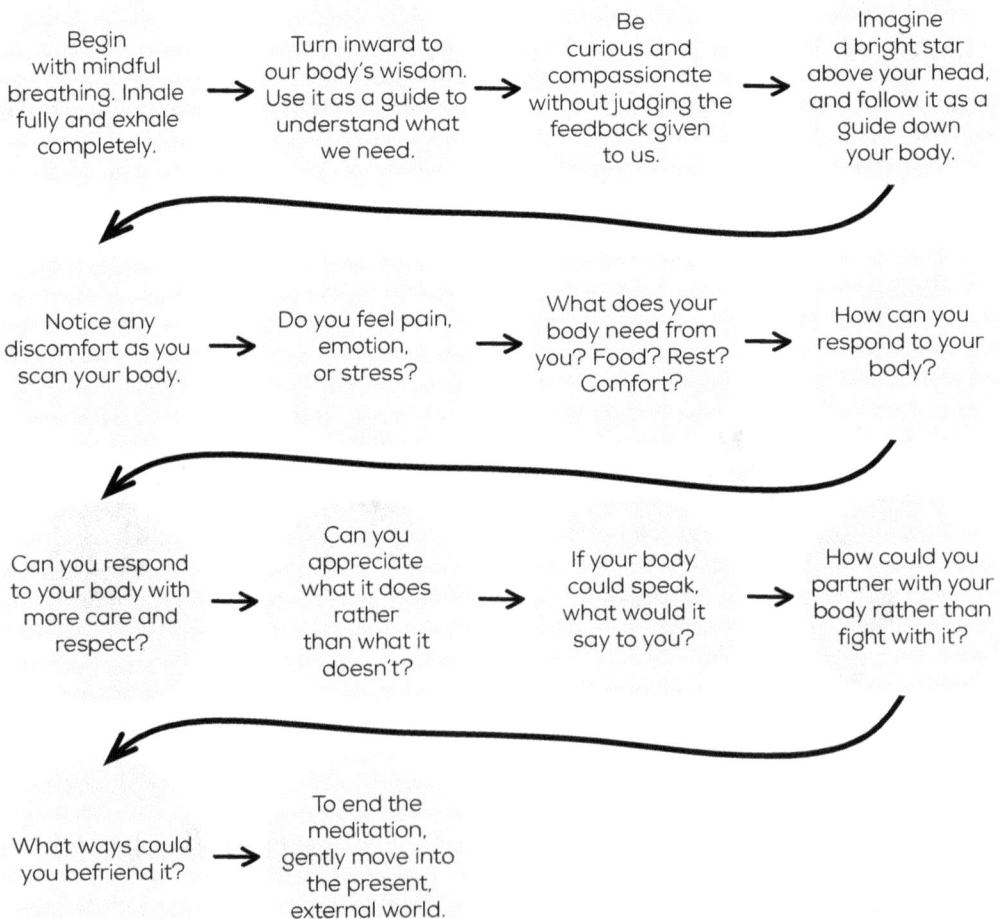

Begin with mindful breathing. Inhale fully and exhale completely. → Turn inward to our body's wisdom. Use it as a guide to understand what we need. → Be curious and compassionate without judging the feedback given to us. → Imagine a bright star above your head, and follow it as a guide down your body.

Notice any discomfort as you scan your body. → Do you feel pain, emotion, or stress? → What does your body need from you? Food? Rest? Comfort? → How can you respond to your body?

Can you respond to your body with more care and respect? → Can you appreciate what it does rather than what it doesn't? → If your body could speak, what would it say to you? → How could you partner with your body rather than fight with it?

What ways could you befriend it? → To end the meditation, gently move into the present, external world.

Return to this meditation often. Notice what you observe in your body.

_____

_____

_____

_____

_____

_____

_____

_____

_____

_____

_____

_____

_____

_____

_____

_____

_____

_____

solution

Mindful Solutions

Safe Place Meditation

You can find safety anytime and anywhere by going on a mini- vacation in your mind. Find a comfortable private spot and begin mindful breathing. Close your eyes if it is safe to do so. Add music or nature sounds, if helpful, to set the mood. Recall someplace you felt completely safe, a place of awe, a time you were in the ventral vagal state.

As you breathe with intention, fully and completely, surround yourself with the memory of all the beautiful sensory input you experienced.

What are you seeing? Notice the colors, the objects, the panorama. Look to the right and left. Are you alone? Are there others nearby or at a distance? Soak in the scene.

Now, add the sense of sound. What are you hearing in this scene? Notice close-up sounds and far away sounds.

Now, add the sense of touch or external feeling. What is the temperature? Is there sunshine, and can you feel it on your skin? Can you feel wind or a light breeze, or is it still? If you are inside, what is the lighting or temperature of the room? What are you standing or sitting on? What does it feel like underneath you? Are you touching anything or anyone and, if so, what is the sensation?

Now, add the sense of smell, which may also prompt the sense of taste in your mouth.

How do you feel in your body? Make sure you are still breathing slowly and deeply. Are you able to find contentment, safety, and calm—if even for a short while?

You did it. This is your safe-place meditation.

Describe your safe place in detail here.

_____

_____

_____

_____

_____

_____

_____

_____

_____

_____

_____

_____

_____

_____

Mindful Solutions

The Wave Meditation

The wave meditation is used to shift or release intense energy or emotion in your body.

Imagine yourself on the edge of the ocean, safe from harm, yet where you can feel the immense volume of water moving in and out from the shoreline. Your bare feet are planted firmly in the sand and it's warm. The sea spray mists you, creating a pleasant temperature in combination with the sunshine. You can smell and taste the salty air.

Place your hands on the area of the most distress and emotional energy in your body, and begin to breathe in and out of that area of your body. Breathe in unison with the waves moving onto the shore and receding out to sea again. As the waves get closer, imagine the discomfort in your body growing in size and intensity. When the waves flow back out to sea, imagine the discomfort getting smaller and less intense. Now, imagine the waves coming even closer and washing over your body. As each wave recedes, imagine it carrying more and more of your discomfort out to sea with it, leaving you firmly planted on the shore. You are feeling less discomfort and much more clarity. The sun, water, and sand have renewed your energy, confidence, and courage.

Write about your experience with this wave meditation.

solution

_____

_____

_____

_____

_____

_____

_____

_____

_____

_____

_____

_____

_____

_____

_____

_____

_____

_____

_____

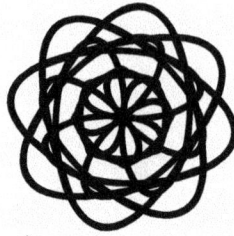

8 C's

Experience

This session will focus on Calm.

"Be Calm"

Draw a picture, symbol, or phrase reminding and anchoring you to the feeling of calm.

Reflect and list moments in your life when you felt calm.

_____

_____

_____

How can you create more calm in your life?

_____

_____

_____

Reflection and Discussion

Reflection: Use this space to reflect on insights gained from this session. What have you learned? What can you implement?

Discussion: For group leaders:

- Ask if anyone, or all, would care to share a story or memory. Tend to feelings.

- Ask the group to share their autonomic ladders or body maps. Encourage curiosity and discussion.

- Discuss "Mindful Solutions" and practice the meditations.

- Discuss the "Self-Care Solutions" and strategies for shifting autonomic states using the senses.

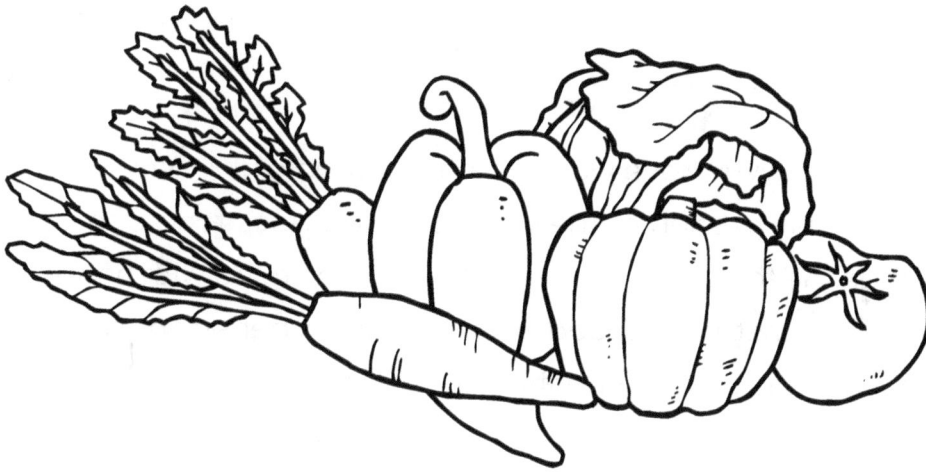

session three

"Eat Food. Not too much. Mostly plants."

Michael Pollan

Nourish

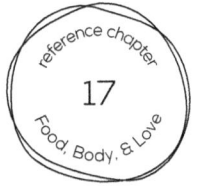

Food is our life force. Why have we become so afraid of it? Why have we made it so complicated? This session of the workbook discusses food and eating. Eating well is more than the food you put on your fork. It has to do with how you think and feel about food. For instance, if food is eaten while experiencing feelings of fear, it creates stress that can offset benefits intended for your transformational journey.

My wish for you is to:

- Approach food with curiosity.
- Feel better each time you have eaten.
- Think of hunger as a gift rather than a burden.
- Feel safe with what and how much food you eat.
- Know food is medicine for the body, heart, and soul.
- Share the pleasure of food in connection with others.
- Develop a collaborative relationship with food that fosters trust between you and your body.

Before we get into the details of eating, let's explore what may have made you feel afraid to eat and feel so out of control with food.

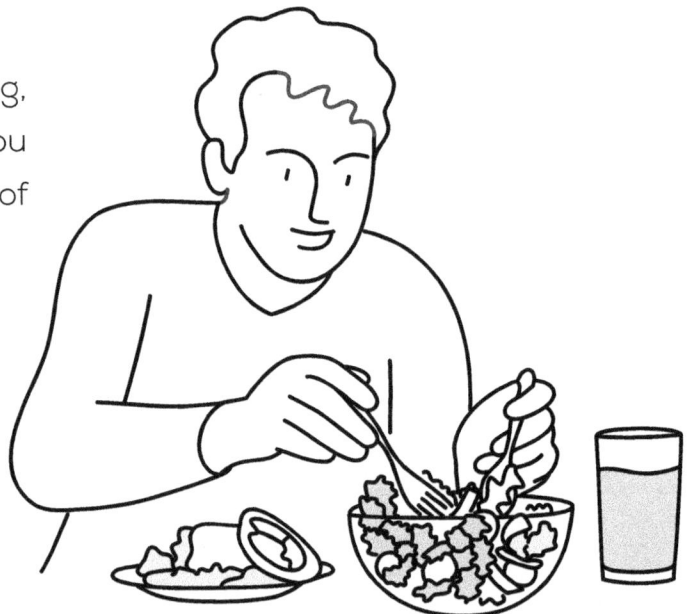

Hunger, Cravings, and Free Will

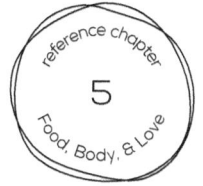

reference chapter 5 *Food, Body, & Love*

Everyone's body and brain has been imprinted with a blueprint/food journey, influencing how you think about and respond to food and eating. The single most influential factor in our feeding behavior is food insecurity. This is the fear of not having enough food, or not being allowed to have as much food as you would like. Nearly every client's story has the thread of food insecurity running through it.

The body has a natural drive to find food for survival, and any threat to this need creates fear. The body doesn't know there is a Costco nearby, it only responds to what it's been fed or not fed, allowed or not allowed. In any relationship that uses control, there is fear. Food restriction nearly always backfires.

It is essential to employ free will when making decisions regarding food. Autonomy and choice disengage fear and rebellion around food choices.

Tell your story of Food Insecurity.

_____

_____

_____

_____

_____

_____

_____

_____

Unravel Diet and Food Rules

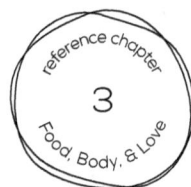

reference chapter

3

Food, Body, & Love

Our eating behaviors are influenced by the diet and food rules we've picked up over the years from well-meaning authority figures, social media fads, and the multibillion-dollar diet or food industry. Most people have a set of beliefs or rules about food and eating. I bet you have a few, and they are likely influencing your food choices and eating behaviors—whether you are aware of them or not.

Without judgment, list some of the internalized rules that may be complicating your relationship with food and eating.

_____

_____

_____

_____

_____

_____

_____

_____

_____

Are you willing to loosen your grip on these beliefs? We often hold a tight fist when we are afraid, rather than lead with a relaxed, open hand. The goal is to observe your beliefs and revisit their origin. If they no longer serve you but feed your fear, it might be time to let them go and move on.

Neutralize Perfectionism

Perfectionism is a common trait among those with troubled eating. When there is little flexibility in eating behavior, it can lead to an "all or nothing" pattern of eating. With the hope of following the rules again someday soon, individuals will eat food they may not be hungry for in preparation for the next diet plan or cycle. These destructive swings are demoralizing. Sometimes our internalized critical voice is so loud, we use food binges to dissociate and numb out. We want to escape and not worry about food for a little while. Unfortunately, we wake up to find we've made things worse.

In this food healing journey, I ask that you take a flexible long-term approach. This is an investment in a long and enduring relationship with your body. Take on a pattern of "mostly and sometimes" when it comes to food and life, understanding perfectionism only leads to suffering and misery.

The Neurobiology of Food Intake Is Complicated

What drives us to eat? Why do we get hungry or crave certain foods? It involves many factors including the brain's reward system, the endocrine system, vagal nerve messaging from the gut, and energy balance signaling. Most of the messaging is beyond our conscious awareness. So, most of our drive to eat is out of our immediate control. Please be compassionate with yourself. If you have tried intuitive eating and loved the freedom from dieting, but found yourself feeling out of control with food, you didn't get the rest of the story. Here it is.

Reward Expectancy and Learning

Your brain has developed a habit of driving you to eat certain foods without you being conscious of it. The culprit is dopamine, the neurotransmitter that establishes pathways for pleasure and reward. We will take a deeper dive into this later in the workbook, but for now, all you need to know is the "want" and obsession you have for certain foods is real. To make matters worse, you may also have difficulty staying present and mindful due to "overloaded" brain circuits. This makes you vulnerable to automatic and habitual impulsivity. In short, you may not be readily able to say "no" when you find yourself in difficult environments. It's not your fault... but there are solutions. There is hope!

Gut Microbiome

Your gut sends signals to your brain via the vagus nerve, called the gut-brain axis. If there is imbalance within your gut *microbiome*–the population of bacteria residing in your gut, your brain may receive signals to eat more refined carbohydrates.

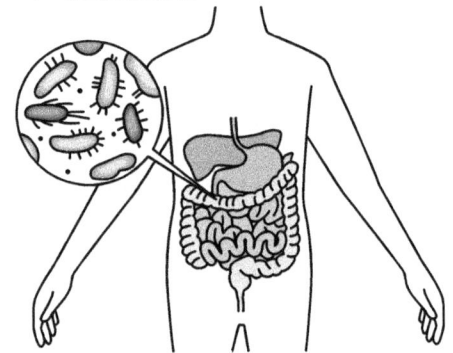

Bacteria within your gut feed on the food we eat to obtain their energy and fuel. When they run out, they dial up for more. Certain types of gut bacteria thrive on sugar to produce hormones that alter our hunger and satiety. These bacteria make us feel uneasy and dissatisfied until their cravings are met. They crowd out and suppress the more helpful bacteria in our gut to maximize their own chances of flourishing. This gut imbalance may be the reason why the more processed food we eat, the more we crave. Crazy, right?

The Blood Sugar and Anxiety Connection

Eating for mental health is a real thing. I would rather help people focus on eating to feel good rather than to manipulate their weight to look good. Do you suffer from chronic anxiety? It could be caused or intensified by a blood sugar imbalance. What we eat effects our mood. When we ingest an imbalanced meal high in sugar or carbohydrates, our blood sugar and insulin levels go up, and we get a surge of energy. This is followed by a sudden drop or crash in blood sugar, taking our energy and mood down with it. So, we go from feeling great to feeling anxious, tired, and irritable. To feel better and get our energy back, we are driven to eat more carbohydrates, and the cycle repeats.

Another example of the blood sugar and anxiety connection is when we go many hours without eating because we fear we'll start bingeing. Going that long without food causes our blood sugar to drop, leaving us feeling anxious and driving us toward our next binge episode. The more stable our blood sugar, the better our mental health, and the fewer our food cravings.

Do you think your anxiety is affected by low blood sugar? Why or why not?

_____

_____

_____

_____

_____

_____

_____

Can you think of some specific times when low blood sugar left you feeling anxious?

_____

_____

_____

_____

_____

_____

_____

_____

_____

_____

_____

_____

_____

_____

_____

_____

_____

A System Reboot

If you are experiencing bingeing or having difficulty with obsessional cravings, my recommendation is to reset your internal eating clock. This is much like resetting your sleep schedule when your sleep cycle is out of synch. For example, if you have a habit of staying up late and sleeping in, the best thing to do is start getting up earlier so you tire earlier and fall asleep at a more desirable time. Painful, I know.

To reset your internal eating clock, you need to eat predictably and dose food throughout the day. This will keep your keep blood sugar levels stable. It will also keep you calm and create feelings of food security. This type of eating, called structured eating, helps reset your hunger and satiety cues. Don't let the word structure bother you or get your defenses up. Remember, where there is no structure, there is chaos and anxiety.

So, eat breakfast within a couple of hours of waking even if you're not hungry for it, and continue to eat 3 predictable meals and a couple of snacks each day, if hungry. Structured eating is one of the best ways to reboot the system!

Another effective way is to eat more whole foods, decrease processed foods, and balance nutrients and food groups. You are going to get a chance to practice that in just a bit, and it's fun!

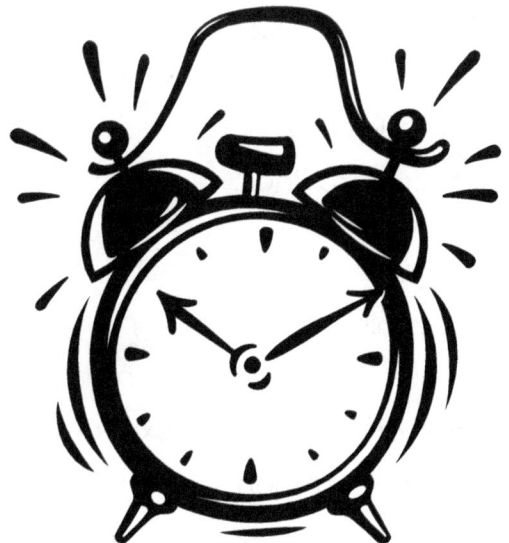

Understanding the Difference Between Hunger and Cravings

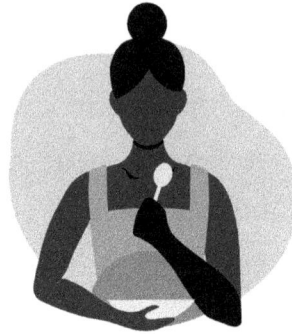

It may be difficult to distinguish between hunger and cravings, but by practicing mindful awareness, you will begin to understand the difference. Both are physical sensations, but my experience is they tend to come from different parts of the body and have a "different language." I have included a Hunger Scale and a Cravings Scale in the "Mindful Solutions" section you can come back to time and time again.

Mindful eating is where we are headed in our journey, and there are certain baby steps needed to get us there. Armed with the body scans we colored in "Session Two," we can pause and pay attention to the internal nervous system states driving us to eat. What cues or triggers may have started the process? Sensory cues such as the sight of food, smell, or the actual act of tasting food starts our brain "talking" to us. It makes us anxious to think of not getting the food. Certain times of the day, or familiar environments associated with food, may be cues for discomfort. These are likely cravings.

Hunger, on the other hand, tends to come with physical symptoms like low energy, foggy thinking, being "hangry," and having an empty feeling or "growling" sensation in your stomach. The interesting frustrating truth is cravings often stimulate symptoms like those experienced with hunger. So, pay attention to meal timing and use common sense in determining the difference. Good luck! Remember to be curious and nonjudgmental throughout this journey.

Food, Fear, and Change

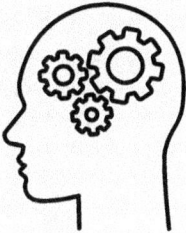

"Lifestyle-based interventions work best when the choices are motivated by an intrinsic drive for vitality and not out of fear."

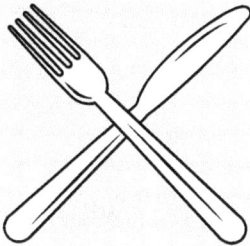

Otherwise, recommending a style of eating or that feels restrictive can cause a rebound into old patterns.

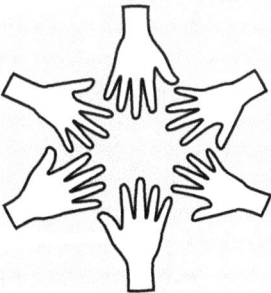

"Our relationship with food is as important as the food we eat."

A Harm Reduction Model of Eating

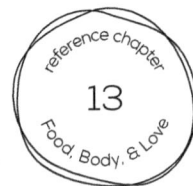

The purpose of harm-reduction eating is to help reboot your neurobiological system so you crave and obsess less over foods. The goal is to feel better physically, have more mental clarity, and feel more in charge of your life. It's important not to make this into another diet that reinforces a restrictive mindset. It is meant to reframe your approach to eating. You are now on a self-care journey for the body and mind.

A harm-reduction model of eating helps the body feel safe and secure. You are being fed predictably, in a nourishing way, without overfeeding it with upsetting, inflammatory foods. Harm reduction is different than abstinence in that we employ the moderate approach of "mostly and sometimes," because life happens, and compassion is key when it comes to caring for yourself.

There are 6 Keys to the Harm-Reduction Model. They will be a vital guide as you begin to reboot your system.

Six Keys

1   Eat three to six times a day, with the first meal/snack in the morning. Find a rhythm that works for you, depending on how much you eat at any one time, what your energy needs are, and how your daily routine is structured. Try to remain flexible and stay curious about what works for you. The goal is to create a safe predictable pattern of eating. Be intentional about your meals and snacks. Sit down, plate it, and make sure meals have a start and finish to them.

2

Using high-fiber nutrient-dense foods (mostly plants), eat to satiety without limitations. This will help decrease cravings while feeding the good bacteria in your gut. Listen to your body with curiosity and respond compassionately. Don't binge but do fill up on whole foods, which are metabolized more slowly than processed foods. Whole foods stick with you longer and are often more satisfying.

3

Balance all your meals and snacks by including a high-quality protein to keep your blood sugar levels stable. Aim for equal portions of protein and complex carbohydrates. Include a source of fats at every meal and snack. These keep your mind and body satisfied, creating an "all is well" feeling. Note: Since fats are calorie-dense, they are eaten in smaller quantities than proteins and complex carbohydrates.

4

Experiment with food choices and eating behaviors that produce intrinsic rewards like physical energy, mental clarity, and the fewest GI disturbances. If this means choosing to remove some items from your diet for a while, like dairy or gluten, reframe your choice as an act of care rather than one of restriction. Make sure you're doing it for the right reasons. Remember it's not about being good, it's about feeling good!

5

Some foods may need to be eaten with more care. These are usually those, delicious, processed foods you once obsessed over or felt out of control with. These are your "cravings foods." Make these your "sometimes" foods, eaten with love in mind. Eat them mindfully,

5
(cont.)

joyfully, and with others while making memories. We want to train the brain that these foods have a place in our lives, but they are not to be eaten habitually for the purpose of escape or to regulate our emotions.

Please do not eat these foods in the spirit of fear. You have self-care solutions and various meditations to help you regulate your nervous system when you feel anxious and afraid. Use them, they are there for you.

I don't know about you, but I ate my cravings food in a manner that was mindless, creating isolation and shame. When you start harm-reduction eating, cravings foods are best kept out of sight and mind, so you are not triggering the brain to crave them. Eventually, they will become your "sometimes" foods, eaten in the spirit of love and connection.

6

Lastly, it's important to monitor yourself for feelings of depletion, scarcity, and rebellion. If they show up, use a few of the self-care solutions to calm yourself. When you become triggered and yield to food out of fear, compassion is key. Take a time out and respond to the feeling with care and love. You may have relied on food for self-regulation and companionship in the past, but you have new solutions at your fingertips. This is a good time to go back to "Session Two" and review the Solutions. They will help you restore calm and a feeling of safety. In other words, they will bring you into a ventral vagal state so important for your health and wellbeing. If you do turn to food, oh well, it's just food; there is no moral judgment there.

Creating Your Owner's Manual for Feeding Yourself

Activity

Having a plan helps you prepare and make mindful choices. This is especially important for those times when you tend to be automated and impulsive, like when you're tired, scattered, and distracted. The key is to create guidelines that direct your choices without having to resort to obsessive rules and perfectionistic tendencies.

The plate planner is one such model. When you get started with this, the idea is to keep it simple. It is probably not the time to try complex, elaborate, recipes. It's more about food assembly: filling plates and bowls, building salads, creating smoothies, and whipping up skillet meals. Plate planning also helps with making shopping lists and streamlining food preparation.

Plate Planner

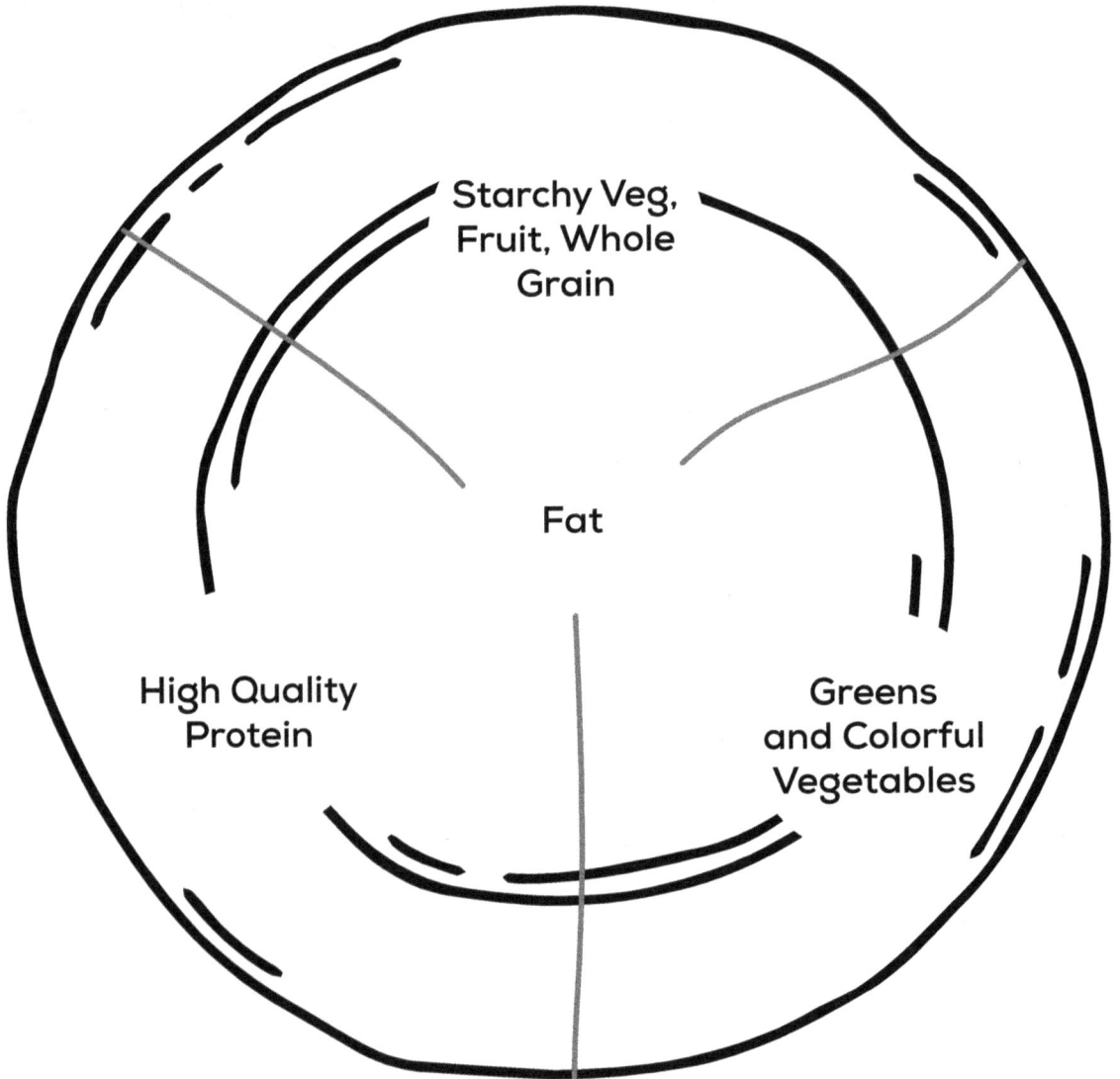

Starchy Veg,
Fruit, Whole
Grain

Fat

High Quality
Protein

Greens
and Colorful
Vegetables

My Foods

To plan great meals, you will first list foods you like in each category. Don't list a food because you think you should eat it. The idea is to build balanced meals out of foods you enjoy! Practice building a few meals by adding one food to your plate for each category. Have fun and be creative.

In putting together your food list of personal preferences, I got the ball rolling for you. Circle those foods you prefer, but feel free to add to the lists.

High-Quality Proteins

Lean Meats
Fish: salmon, tuna, shrimp, cod
Chicken: breasts, thighs, tenders
Turkey: breasts, lunch meat
Beef: roast beef slices
Pork: chops, loin

Eggs

Low-fat Dairy or
Unsweetened Dairy Substitutes
High protein yogurt
Hard and soft cheeses
Cottage cheese
Kefir
Soy milk
Whey protein powder

Plant-Based Proteins
Pea protein powder
Nuts or nut butter
Firm tofu
Tempeh, Lentils, Quinoa
Plant-based burgers

Other: List

_____

_____

_____

_____

_____

_____

_____

_____

_____

_____

_____

Complex Carbohydrates

Starchy Vegetables
Potatoes: baked, sweet
Squash: acorn, butternut, spaghetti
Corn
Peas

Beans and Legumes
Pinto, black, garbanzo
Black-eyed peas,
Bean Pasta
Lentils

Grain, whole
Quinoa, barley, oats, brown rice,
cous-cous, whole-grain pasta,
whole-grain bread

Fruits, whole
Apple, pear, pineapple, grapes,
citrus, berries

Other: List

_____

_____

_____

_____

_____

_____

_____

_____

_____

_____

_____

Greens and Rainbow of Vegetables
(fresh, frozen, fermented)

Greens
Leafy greens; cabbage, lettuce, kale,
spinach, bok choy

Rainbow
Onion, garlic, shallots, carrots,
celery, cucumber, peppers,
green beans, cauliflower (whole/
riced), broccoli

Other: List

_____

_____

_____

_____

_____

Fats

Plant-based
Nuts and seeds, butters and oils
Avocado, avocado oil
Olives, olive oil
Spray oils

Animal-based
Butter, mayonnaise, sauces and
dressings, dips
Dark chocolate
Cheese

Other: List

_____

_____

_____

_____

_____

_____

_____

_____

After purchasing these items, store them in the pantry, freezer, or refrigerator grouped by food lists. This makes it easy to select from each group when building meals. If food preparation is a hassle or time concern, buy foods ready to add, zap, or heat without much thought. Remember to make things easy to grab and assemble without hesitation. The brain will talk you out of something if it isn't easy.

Cook your grains or proteins ahead, or buy them already cooked, and store in glass containers. You want to be able to see what you have with one quick glance. If you like adding vegetables to your creations, buy them already chopped, or chop them and store in glass containers. If you like adding beans, empty the can, rinse and drain the beans, and store them in glass containers. If you store your fruits and vegetables in plastic bags in the bottom drawer, you will forget about them, and they will die alone in the dark. Put items you want to snack on at eye level. Make it easy.

So How Much Do I Eat?

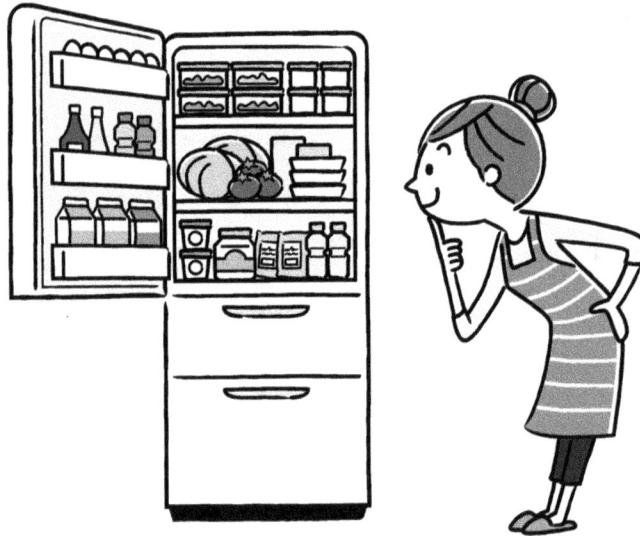

Create and arrange your plates, bowls, skillets, salads, and smoothies with the Plate Planner in mind rather than worry about precise portion sizes. The balance of proteins to carbohydrates is important for keeping your blood sugar stable. To ensure your food is tasty and satisfying, remember to include fats on your plate whether they are added to the food (like olive oil), are in the food (natural fat in beef), or are used as part of the meal (sliced avocado). Now, create some plates, bowls, skillets, salads and smoothie meals to get started. Make sure to include a couple of Comfort Meals for when you need that full feeling. (You know what I mean.)

Write a menu on plates using your food lists for each section of the plate.

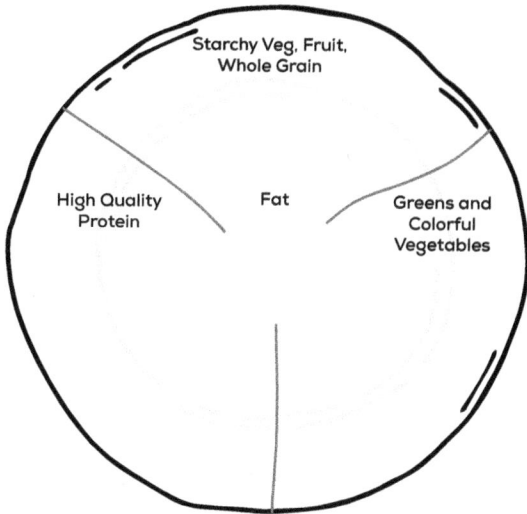

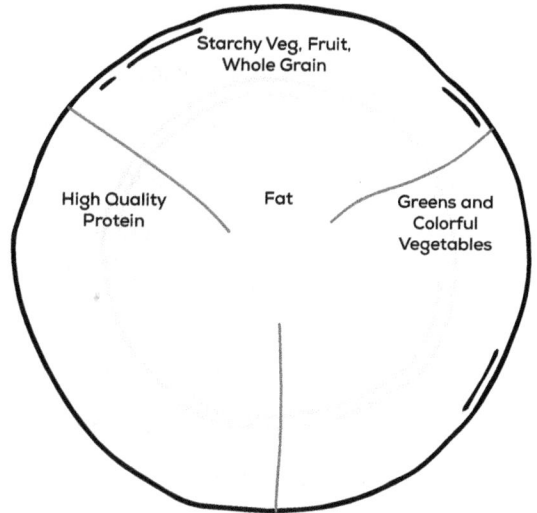

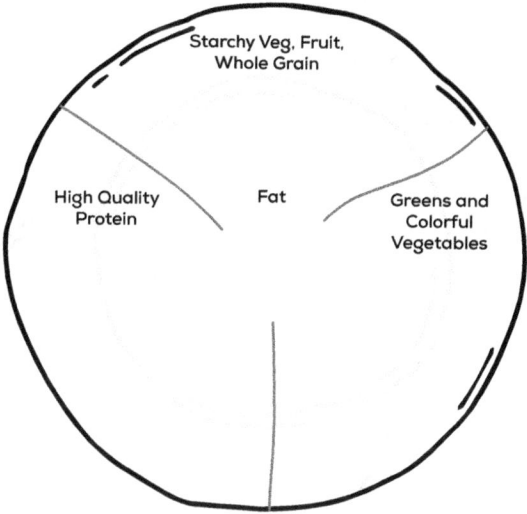

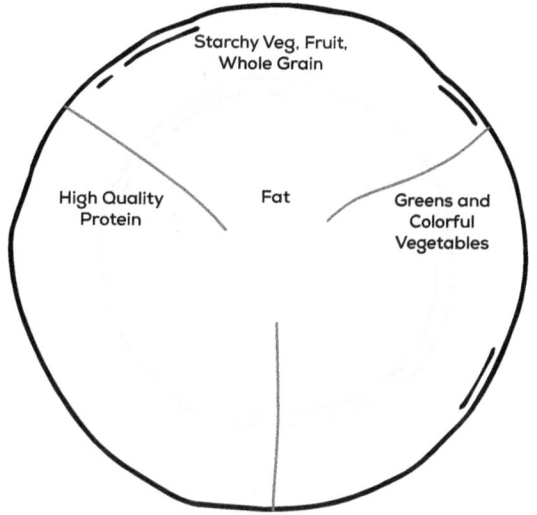

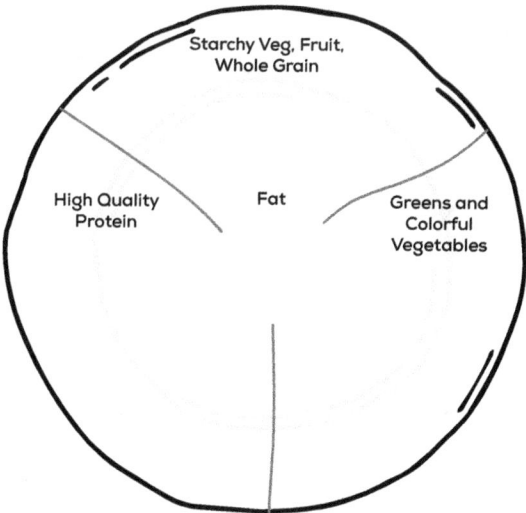

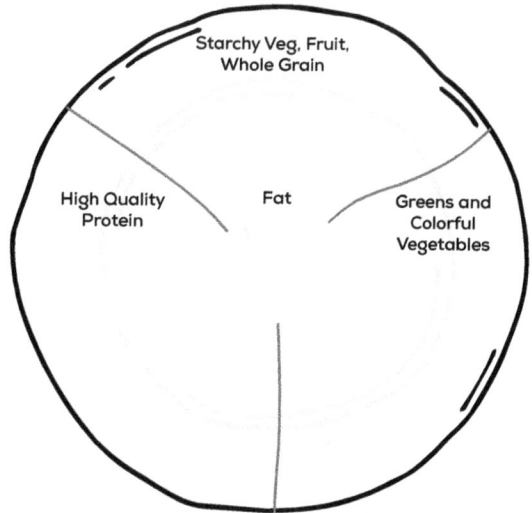

Now create some easy snacks ideas: things that can be kept with you or at your workplace, or something at eye level in the refrigerator or pantry. Snacks are not a dinner plate but rather a bread plate. The best snacks include a balance of protein, complex carbs, and a fat to make it more satisfying. Some proteins options have enough fat in them, no need for extra fat.

Here are a few examples of balanced snacks:
- Hummus and sliced raw veggies
- Chicken left from last night's dinner, a cheese stick, and an apple
- Peanut butter and celery sticks
- Deli turkey, a slice of cheese, and a few crackers
- A hard-boiled egg, a piece of fruit, and a few almonds

What snack combinations can you create using a protein, complex carb, and a fat?

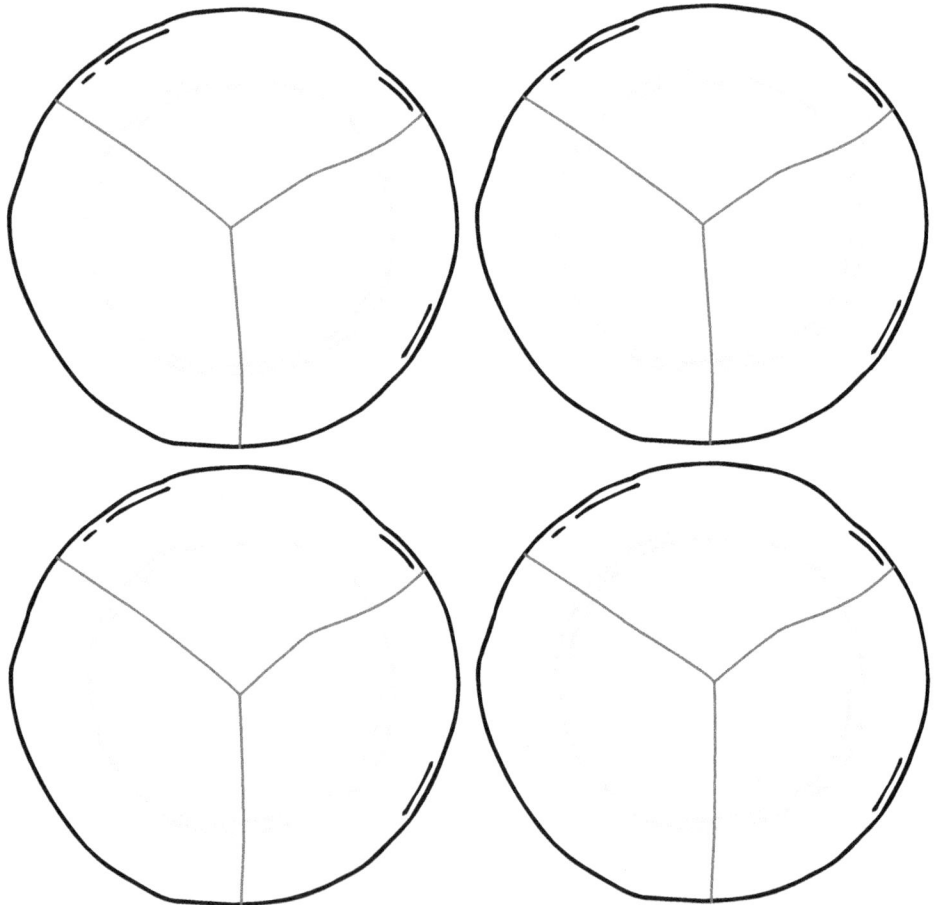

"Hey? What about eating out?" Great question. Spend some time looking at menus from your favorite restaurants and find items you could order to "build" a balanced plate. For example, you might decide on chicken Caesar salad. The grilled chicken is a protein, the salad provides the greens, dressing adds the necessary fat, and the croutons round out the criteria for carbs.

List the restaurants and menu items you could use to build balanced, tasty meals. This way, you'll be prepared when you are feeling spontaneous or when family and friends come to call.

Restaurant   *Order*

"This all feels super healthy and "diet-y." What about Fun Foods?" Take a breath. Let's revisit why you are doing this. This reboot is about care and healing of the body and retraining the brain. The purpose is for you to begin feeling less controlled by food, to be more in charge and work in collaboration with your body. If you want a treat or a processed comfort meal, here is the suggested process:

Treat Treats like Treats

1. Make sure you are not starving. Take the edge off first with one of your snack options.

2. Make sure it's a treat you love. Don't settle for just any treat. If you want a cookie or ice cream, make sure it's your favorite.

3. Make sure you are with others, connecting and making joyful memories.

4. Eat mindfully and stay present. Savor the taste and enjoy the richness of the experience.

5. There is no place for guilt. You chose this experience, enjoy it. Move on to your plate planner for your next meal or snack.

6. We want to make pleasant memories with these foods rather than experience them in secret or use them to manage stress or pain.

"I'm afraid I'll lose control, and I won't stop once I start eating." You may need some *exposure work* and brain training activities around food "cravings." That activity is next up!

Brain Training for Addressing Cravings

Activity

Adapted from Dr. Boutelle UCSD research on binge eating

Preparation

1. Do not do this activity if you are hungry or thirsty. If you are hungry or thirsty, get a small snack or drink before starting the exposure.

2. For the exposure, choose a food you typically crave that makes you feel out of control once you start eating it. Only prepare a small snack plate of this food. Don't purchase a lot of this food or store it in your home. Some choose to go out for this exposure and have someone around for support.

3. Be prepared to document your answers to the questions as you go through this activity with me, step by step. Review the Craving Scale in the Solutions section of this session, you'll be asked to reference it often.

4. The total exposure should be at least five minutes. You can repeat this with another food if you like, but don't do more than three food exposures in one session.

5. When you eat these foods outside of the exposure activity, make sure to eat them slowly and mindfully while connecting with others and making happy memories. These foods are not "bad." We are helping to train your brain not to crave them.

Pre-Assignment

1. How much are you craving the food in front of you right now? (Use rating scale.)

2. What is the highest level of craving you think you will experience during this exposure?

3. If you could eat as much as you wanted, how much do you think you would eat right now? (1=none and 5=all of it)

4. How hard do you think the exposure to this food will be? (1=easy and 5=very difficult)

5. How confident are you that you can resist your urge to eat during the exposure activity today? (1= low and 5=high)

_____

_____

_____

Assignment

1. Pick up the exposure food, hold it in your hands, and rate your craving.

2. Notice the thoughts in your head when you look at the food.

3. Take a big whiff of the food and rate your craving. What do you notice about the color, texture, smell, and feeling of the food you are holding in your hand?

4. Now, take one small bite, or taste of the food, and rate your craving.

5. What sensations do you notice in your stomach or other parts of your body when you focus on the food? Do you notice yourself salivating?

6. Notice the taste of the food in your mouth. Notice if you want more of the food, and rate your craving.

7. Put the food down, if you haven't already, and rate your craving. Do you notice any other urges?

8. Now, pick up the food as though you were going to take a bite of it. Imagine how it will taste, without eating it. Rate your craving.

9. Think about the last time you ate this food.

10. Take a big whiff of the food and rate your craving.

11. Keep taking big whiffs and think about how pleasant or unpleasant it smells.

12. Now, take a small bite, or taste of the food and rate your craving.

13. Does this food remind you of other foods or situations?

14. Notice the taste of the food in your mouth. Notice if you want more and rate your craving.

15. Put the food down and rate your craving now.

16. Think about the last time you ate this food. Who were you with? What did it taste like? How much did you eat?

17. Make your final craving rating now.

18. Throw this food in the trash, or get it out of sight.

_____

_____

_____

_____

Post-Assignment

1. How much do you crave the food now?

2. What was the highest level of craving you experienced during the exposure?

3. If the food was in front of you right now, how much do you think you would eat? (1=none and 5=all of it)

4. How hard was resisting the food during the exposure? (1=easy and 5= very difficult)

5. How confident do you feel now about resisting your cravings or urges to eat this food in real life? (1= easy and 5=very difficult)

6. Write any additional comments.

_____

_____

_____

_____

_____

_____

_____

_____

_____

Mindful Solutions

Hunger vs. Cravings Scales

Craving Scale

5   **Explosive** – I don't care. I want it. I cannot resist the food, no matter how hard I try.

4   **Strong** – I really want it. It's hard not to think about it. My concentration is impaired as I plot and plan to get the food.

3   **Moderate** – Wow, that food looks good. I wish I had some.

2   **Somewhat** – That food looks good, but I'm going to do other things.

1   **Under Control** – I'm more interested in what I'm doing than having food. I can stay focused and not think about food.

Hunger Scale

5   **Stuffed** – I feel uncomfortable, tired, and lethargic.

4   **Satisfied** – I am energetic and alert. (Note that it usually takes twenty minutes to feel this way.)

3   **Neutral** – I've taken the edge off hunger. I have more energy, but I could eat more.

2   **Hungry** – My stomach is gently growling and feels empty. I'm a little low on energy.

1   **Starving** – My stomach hurts; my head hurts. I'm weak and jittery.

solution

Mindful Solutions

Food is our life force vitality. Move toward food with awe and wonder. Diminish scarcity

Abundance Meditation

This meditation is helpful for those who identify with having food insecurity, we discussed this earlier in this session.

Start breathing in fully and exhaling completely in a natural rhythm that brings feelings of safety. Repeat these words to yourself:

There is always enough food, there is always more. I am in charge now, it's my choice.

If I get hungry, I can always have more food. I have enough, I will always have enough. I can relax now. I have enough, there is always enough for me. I can be assured I can always have more. I only need what I need; I don't have to overcompensate for the scarcity of the past. I never have to go hungry or feel restricted again. I'm in charge, it's my choice. There is more than enough. I can relax into the idea that food will be there the very next time I am hungry. Food is abundant.

What words will you use to remind yourself you are safe and have enough?

_____

_____

_____

Self-Care Solution

Sleep

The sun governs light and darkness, establishing our biological rhythms and setting our internal master clock. One of the most basic of life's rhythms is our sleep-wake cycle. Sleep, as you know, is the foundation of health. During sleep, damaged cells are repaired, and our energy is restored.

If we have poor sleep, our health is compromised. Our memory, our immune system, regulation of our appetite, the assimilation of nutrients into energy for repair, the production of neurotransmitters, and more, are adversely affected. We were made to spend about a third of our life sleeping. Don't fight it, embrace it!

Establish a consistent routine of winding down and shutting off. Create an ideal sleep environment without the distractions of light, sound, or extreme temperatures. If you have a sleep disorder or suspect one, make it a priority to get help. There are solutions for sleep apnea and insomnia, some you may have never heard of.

What steps can you take to create a better sleep routine and environment?

_____

_____

_____

_____

_____

_____

If sleep is a serious problem, who will you reach out to for help with solutions?

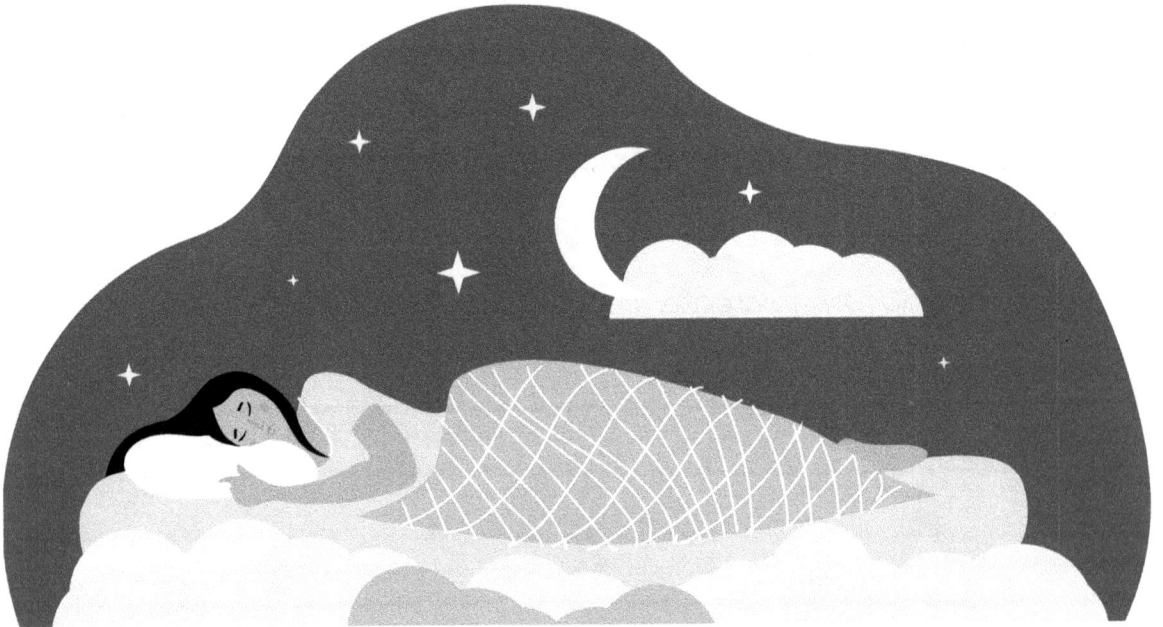

_____

_____

_____

_____

_____

_____

_____

8 C's

Experience

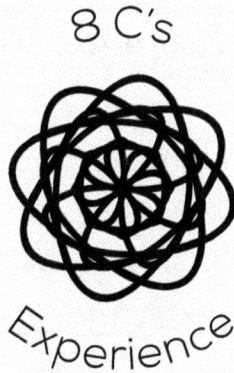

In this session we will focus on Curiosity.

"Be Curious"

Being curious is a non-judgmental process that opens your mind to exploration and experimentation. Curiosity requires an open mind, without fear of consequences. Curiosity involves taking risks and pushing through fixed mindsets. Being curious helps us overcome fear-based living.

What could you be more curious about?

_____

_____

_____

What keeps you from being more curious?

_____

_____

_____

How could you be more curious about food?

_____

_____

_____

Reflection and Discussion

Reflection: Space for free writing on this chapter's insights

_____

_____

_____

_____

_____

_____

_____

_____

_____

_____

_____

_____

_____

_____

_____

_____

_____

_____

_____

Discussion and Activities for Group Leaders

- Ask if anyone would care to share a story of food insecurity.

- Lead group through a brain training for addressing cravings activity and process.

- Discuss what a harm-reduction model of eating means to each participant.

- Share ideas for meal or snack planning.

- Lead group through an abundance meditation and process.

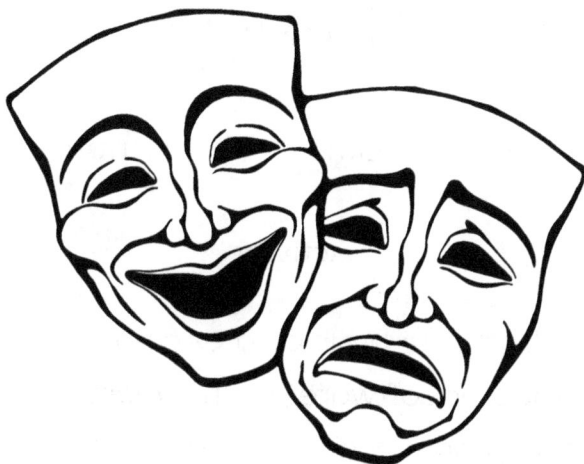

session four

"Perfect Love Casts Out Fear"

1 John 4:18

The Faces of Fear

"OUR PATTERNS OF PROTECTION"

Activity

When we feel fear in our body, our brain creates a narrative to explain it. Our brain is influenced by its "computer software" or the years of programming we have received. Because of this programming, we've developed habitual reactions to fear in an effort to protect ourselves. This helps us feel better and less vulnerable. These protective responses may have been necessary out of survival at one time, but they may not be required or helpful anymore. Let's explore.

The three fear states, as explained by the polyvagal theory, are Fight, Flight, and Freeze. Each state can manifest in different ways. In this activity, we will take a closer look at some of the many faces of fear.

On the next page, circle the words you resonate with for each fear state. Add others as you think of them. Try to approach this from a place of nonjudgment. After all, we are all just trying to manage the best we can. The purpose of this session is to understand our fear responses and, with practice over time, transform them into more positive, productive responses. Doing so requires self-love, self-compassion, and self-acceptance.

We'll do almost anything to avoid the discomfort of fear.
We'll take on many coping strategies to try and manage or
extinguish our fear.

Fight

Chronic anger, defensiveness, control tactics, manipulation, arguing, jealousy, rebellion, self-sabotage, self-abuse including eating disorders, other...

Flight

Procrastination, perfectionism, avoidance, denial, people pleasing, overworking, over exercising, other...

Freeze

Hiding, dissociating, isolating, over-sleeping, numbing and escaping with addiction, bingeing on TV, gaming, or food. deeming oneself unlovable (chronic shame), other...

These patterns of protection take over and hide our authentic self and the gifts we have access to when we are in the ventral vagal state. Fear begets fear, which may explain why you may be stuck in a chronic fear cycle. Your reactions to fear may have served you well in the past, maybe even allowed you to survive horrific trauma or the paralyzing fear of abandonment. Yet, you may not need these "protectors" anymore, and they have simply become chronic habits of fear. It may be time to befriend them and transform them through the calming methods of compassion and love. As I mentioned earlier in this workbook, you may benefit from seeing a trauma specialist to help you through this.

Now take a look at the authentic self and the gifts of the ventral vagal. Circle the words that represent unique parts of yourself and transfer to the map.

Authentic Self   Compassionate, Creative, Confident, Curious, Courageous, Clear, Calm, Connected, Kind, Encouraging, Gifts of Service, Leadership, Lover, Other...

Mapping Your Protective Process

Transfer the words you circled or added onto the map of your protective process on next page.

This provides a visual of why you may be stuck in patterns of protection.

Be patient with your protective parts. Don't judge. Walk alongside your parts and remember they are just trying to keep you safe. Your fear has a long memory. Befriend fear and transform your protective parts with compassion and love. Be a loving parent or friend to your fear.

Fight

Flight

Authentic
Self

Freeze

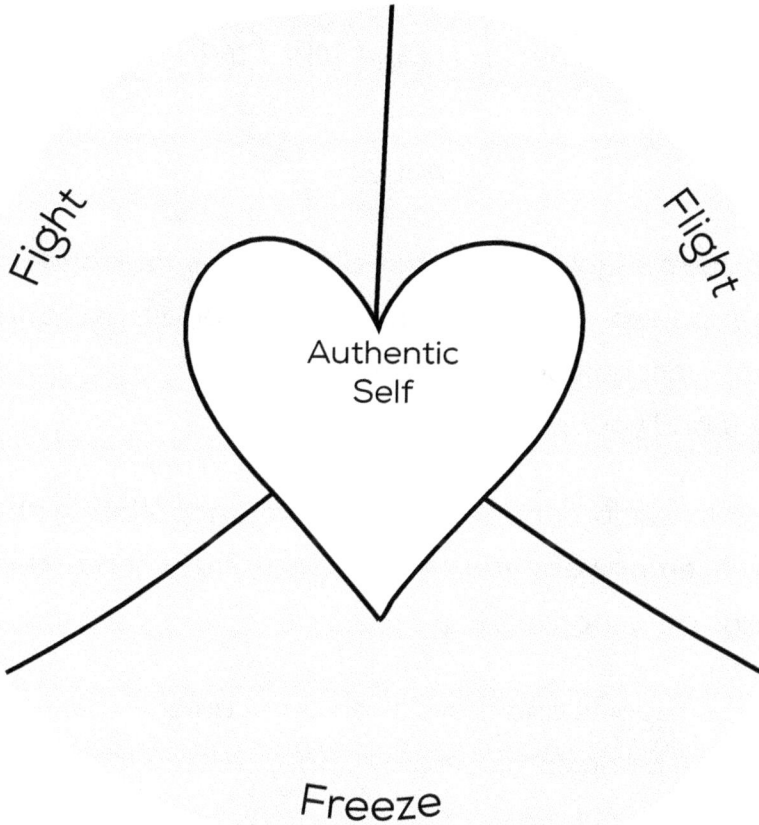

Adapted from Boundaries for Your Soul, Cook & Miller

Let's take some time to reflect on fear. Now that you see your map, are there any surprises? What might happen if you weren't in a state of self-protection?

_____

_____

_____

_____

_____

_____

_____

Love Letters from God

Activity

Love Letters is a form of journaling that disengages fear and imparts wisdom. It calls on a higher power—God, if that fits for you—or a trusted friend, parent, or someone who has unconditional love and regard for you. Someone who knows your authentic self and your potential.

Love Letters uses validation and truth to help you negotiate with your protective parts—your fear. It empowers you to lead your life without defaulting to your protective patterns or responses.

First, express your struggles and fears, then listen quietly. Allow the words to flow through your pen as if being comforted by God, a trusted friend, or perfect parent.

The format goes like this....

Dear _____.

Dear _____.

Of course....you...

What you need to know...

Love, _____

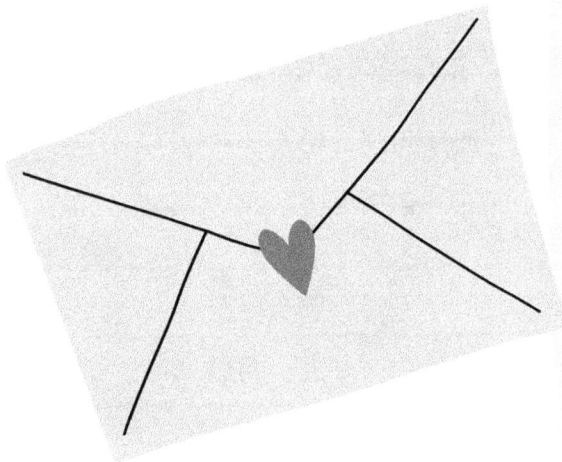

Here is a sample Love Letter to God, and God's response.

Dear Lord,

This has been a hard day. I felt so incompetent and judged today, so exposed to the cruelty of life. I froze, I was speechless. I wanted to fight back, but I didn't. I just stood there and took it all. My insides ached. I couldn't stand it. I counted the minutes until I could be alone to eat and fade away into the blaring sound of the TV. It didn't matter what I ate, I just needed to chew on something and swallow until my insides ached from being full of food instead of aching from feeling like a complete failure. Will I ever be released from the stronghold of food as the answer to all my problems?

My precious Kari,

Of course, you are feeling discouraged. I know it was hard for you today. I know it feels like the ache in your body will never end, but give yourself time to breathe and recover. Count the minutes until you can be alone with me, and I'll give you rest and peace of mind. What you need to know is I love you. Before you even begin to call on me, I am already there cheering you on. You are precious in my eyes; strong, and capable. You will never be alone and will always be safe in my care.

Love, God

This may be a difficult assignment. Perhaps no one has ever spoken to you with such kindness. It can feel awkward and scary to embrace such love and support. Press in. Allow love and compassion to flow over you. These letters, when practiced over and over, can melt the fear and allow you to step into your authentic self.

You can also write letters from your fearful parts and answer from your authentic self. With repetition over time, your fearful parts will retreat to allow your authentic self to lead. In your writing, always start with validation. Validation disengages fear and allows us hear what the other is saying. For example, "I understand because…" We may not agree, but we can find a nugget of relatable truth in each other's story. Practice creates new neuropathways. Keep writing!

Dear _____.

Dear _____.

Of course…you…

What you need to know…

Love, _____

Dear _____

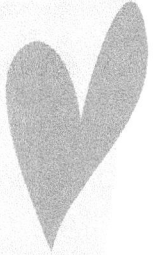

Dear _____

Of course...you...

What you need to know...

Love, _____

Dear _____.

Dear _____.

Of course...you...

What you need to know...

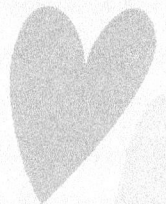

Love, _____

Dear _____

Dear _____

Of course...you...

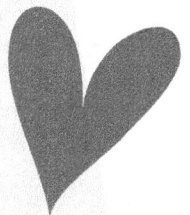

What you need to know...

Love, _____

Mindful Solutions

Compassion

Compassion motivates us to go out of our way to alleviate the physical, mental, and emotional pains of others and ourselves. It allows us to see our own and others' humanity.

Compassion, Latin for "co-suffering," allows for a sensitivity toward the suffering of self and others. It enlists the qualities of patience, wisdom, kindness, perseverance, warmth, and resolve.

Think of a time when you were suffering physically, mentally, or emotionally but neglected to be compassionate with yourself. Now, step back and see yourself through the lens of compassion. Now how might you respond differently?

_____

_____

_____

_____

_____

_____

_____

_____

_____

Mindful Solutions

Meditation and contemplative prayer are methods of extracting fear from our body and bolstering our ventral vagal state. Learning to meditate can shift your mood by re-setting your physical state through visualization. Our brain responds to what is real, as well as what is perceived or visualized.

Infinite Sea of Love Meditation

Begin with mindful breathing. Breathe in fully and exhale completely, using your belly to engage your diaphragm. Take deep belly breaths in and use big sighs to exhale your breath from your lungs. Once comfortably breathing in and out, begin your visualization.

Imagine yourself floating on an infinite sea without a care in the world. Transfixed in the moment, you find yourself bathing in the calm, warm, turquoise waters of a sea of love. The water is buoyant and holds you up, so there is no fear of going under. You float easily, gently rocking, feeling soothed and safe. A white light rises over you and dances off the ripples in the water. There is a sweet smell of flowers in the air swirling around you. You are all alone, but you are not afraid; you feel love all around you.

Completely relaxed, you feel the white light energy surround you and you begin to bring it into your body. Inhale the light of love into your body and exhale any fear that remains. Do several rounds of cleansing inhalations and exhalations. Feel love energy fill your body and trickle into every cell. Notice, or imagine, the thrill of excitement in your heart as you realize this love is unconditional, infinite, and always available to you. Let go of any remaining fear, past or present. Every cell is filled with love.

You are loved, loveable, and safe. This love casts out all fear and any perceived threat. As you go on your way today, you are protected and recharged. You carry this love with you. Others feel love radiating from you, and you can give love freely. Return to this sea of love visualization often to restore calm and expel any fear you pick up along your journey.

Adapted from The Visualizations of The Gabriel Method

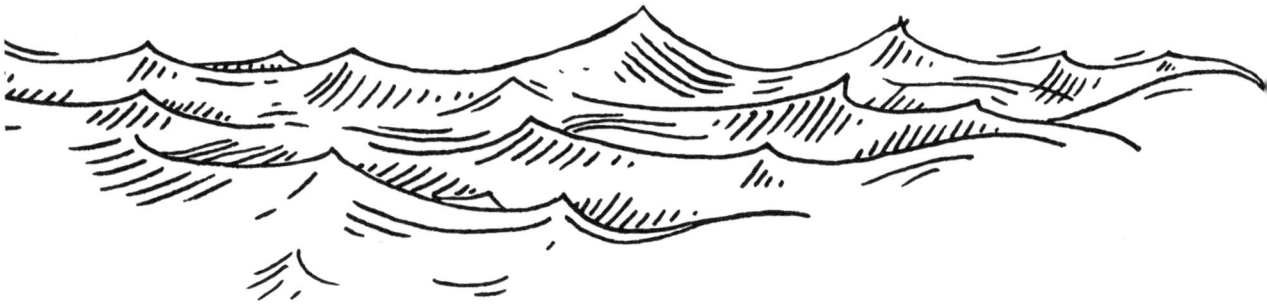

8 C's

Experience

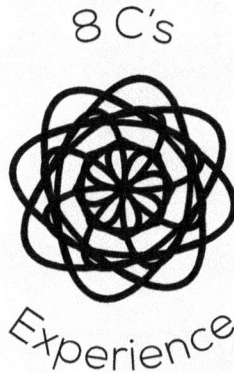

In this session we will focus on Compassion.

"Be Compassionate"

Draw a picture, symbol, or phrase reminding and anchoring you to the feeling of compassion.

Reflect and list the compassionate acts you have received from others in the past. How have you shown compassion toward others? In what ways can you be more compassionate towards yourself?

_____

_____

_____

_____

_____

Reflection and Discussion

Reflection: Use this space to write freely about insights you've gained from this chapter.

_____

_____

_____

_____

_____

_____

_____

_____

_____

_____

_____

_____

_____

_____

_____

_____

_____

Discussion: For group leaders:

- Lead a discussion on the many Faces of Fear.

- Remind the group we all have protective behaviors, most of which have served us well. Discuss behaviors that have worked well in the past but no longer serve us. Instill the idea of befriending and transforming through compassion. Let others share their map of protection.

- Ask if anyone would like to share their love letters.

- Encourage participation and tend to feelings.

- Lead the group in the Sea of Love Meditation.

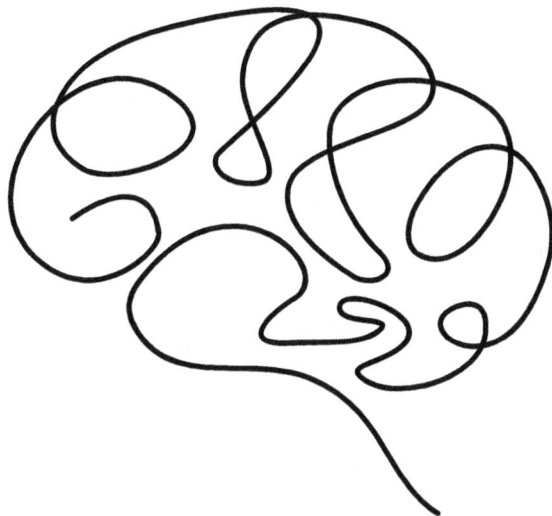

session five

"Our life is what our thoughts make it."

Marcus Aurelius

The Power of Mindset

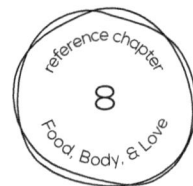

Our thoughts are constant. The brain keeps working and producing thoughts even if we don't want it to. It's a computer, run by software to create a mindset that influences how you feel about yourself, others, and the world around you. Your mindset influences your daily decisions and your life's story. So, if you want to change your story, or life's narrative, you simply need to change the software in your brain.

Is it possible to consciously—by choice—alter our thoughts, attitudes, and beliefs to transform our life and change our future? Absolutely. The brain does not distinguish between an intensely imagined experience and a real one. Athletes have been using visualization for years. An aerial freestyle ski jumper in our last Olympics rehearsed her flips and twists in her mind before pushing off from her platform. She won the gold medal.

We can alter the software running our brain by changing our mindset. Research on the use of placebos gives us proof. Research suggests that the effectiveness of antidepressant medications can be influenced by the placebo effect. In one study, the group that received a placebo or "dummy pill," but thought they were receiving an antidepressant, reported feeling less depressed than the group who did not receive any pills. The fact that the first group members believed they were given the medication somehow changed their physiology enough to improve their mood. That is an example of the placebo effect.

Another study involved an experimental group comprised of housekeepers working for a hotel chain. The sole intervention was they had to attend a lecture on fitness. They were told that the muscles they worked and the cardiovascular fitness they derived from working at their jobs was equal to working out at a gym for several hours a day. It was suggested they were athletes. The control group did not get the lecture. They were not told they were athletes from getting a great workout at their job. The results: those who attended the lecture significantly increased their muscle mass percentage and decreased their blood pressure in four short weeks. It's not magic, it's mindset! You become who and what you think you are.

Who do you think you are? Have you labeled yourself right into a chronic disorder? Many of my clients tell me they are binge eaters. I quickly correct them and say, "You are not a binge eater. You have a habit of bingeing on food for many good reasons." If you are going to take on an identity, take one that promotes the outcomes you want to produce, like the housekeeper athletes. I like to think of myself as a writer. What do writers do every day? They write, of course.

Look at this mindset cycle.

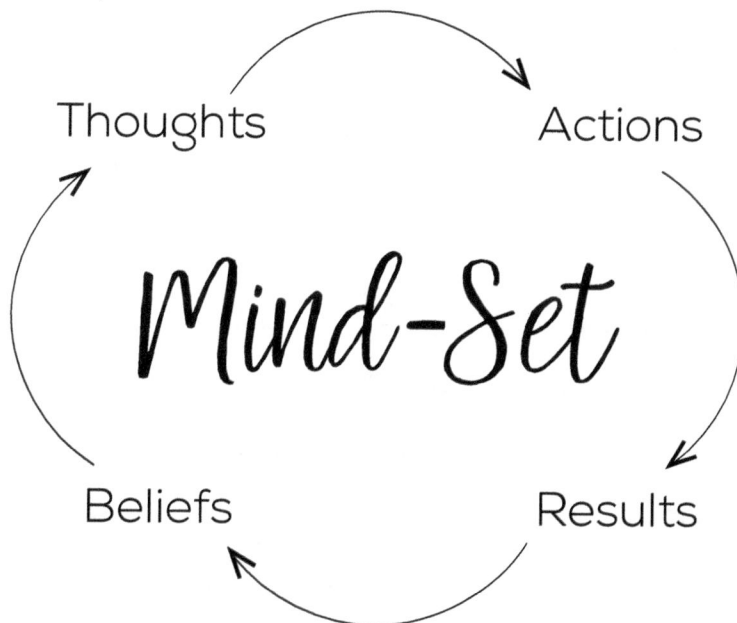

Thoughts → Actions

Mind-Set

Beliefs ← Results

Be careful what you think about and call yourself! Our beliefs and thoughts drive our actions, leading to the results we get in life. That is what is called a self-fulfilling prophecy.

Assignment

Which of your labels or beliefs may have impacted your life's direction?

_____

_____

_____

_____

_____

_____

_____

Which of your strengths, interests, or desires could you leverage to bring you more positive outcomes?

_____

_____

_____

_____

_____

_____

Sticky Brains

Our brain is aware of a thought, emotion, sensation, or image about every fifty milliseconds. It's impossible to stop our brain from thinking, but we can prevent our brain from "sticking."

Some people have very sticky brains. I imagine yellow sticky notes with thoughts pasted inside their brain. They carry a burden of annoying and intrusive thoughts that can nearly drive them mad. The key is to *stop* trying to *stop* them. I learned a term in my doctoral program, *psychojudo*. The premise of this martial-art-of-the-mind is to never strike the thoughts, but rather allow their own energy to direct themselves out of your path. The more you fight the thoughts, the stickier they get.

Using the mindfulness technique of observing and noticing, without attaching or judging, is key. Those with Obsessive Compulsive Disorder are best served by noticing and saying, "Thank you OCD for trying to help me, but next thought please," or "Thank you, and..." It is important to remember many of your thoughts are not true, so don't judge yourself for thinking them. Many are just random ideas, that's all. Bizarre sometimes, but no need to fret. I tell my clients to think of their thoughts as rowdy kids in the backseat of the car. Focused parents can tune them out and keep their eyes on the road. The rowdy kids in the backseat are like thoughts: they are not in charge, and they don't know what's best for them.

So, take charge of the direction you're going, and follow the GPS guided by your values. (More on values in a bit.) If your mind tells you to pull into McDonalds after dropping your real kids off at school, thank it for the suggestion and stay on course.

Let's write some bothersome sticky scripts and practice saying, "Thank you. Next."

Example: Thank you, worry thought, about my body size, I'm choosing to focus on my health and wellbeing.

Thank you, sticky thought (describe) _____

and (value statement) _____

Thank you _____

and _____

Thank you _____

and _____

Thank you _____

and _____

Thank you _____

and _____

Defining Values

Goals vs. Values

Goals give us a target but are future-oriented and dependent on striving..."Are we there yet?"

Once we get "there," we need another goal to keep us happy. Goals define our achievements and what we do.

Values can be lived in each moment. They guide our decisions and are aligned with our most authentic self. They give meaning to who we are and why we are here.

Activity

Circle those values that resonate with you, or add and circle your own at the bottom.

1. Acceptance: to be open to a new view of myself, others, life, etc.

2. Adventure: to actively seek, create, or explore novel or stimulating experiences

3. Agency: to choose how I live and behave, and help others do likewise. To be self-supportive and choose my own way of doing things.

4. Assertiveness: to respectfully stand up for my rights and request what I want

5. Authenticity: to be genuine and real, true to myself

6. Beauty: to appreciate, create, nurture, or cultivate splendor in myself, others, the environment, etc.

7. Caring: to be considerate, compassionate, and gentle toward myself, others, the environment, etc.

8. Challenge: to keep inspiring and motivating myself to grow, learn, and improve

9. Compassion: to act with kindness toward myself and those who are suffering

10. Conformity: to be respectful and obedient of rules and obligations

11. Connection: to engage fully in whatever I am doing; be fully present with others

12. Contribution: to give, help, assist, or make a positive difference for myself or others

13. Cooperation: to work in harmony and collaboration with others

14. Courage: to be brave; to persist in the face of fear, threat, or difficulty

15. Creativity: to be imaginative, innovative, and expressive

16. Curiosity: to be open-minded and interested; to explore and discover

17. Encouragement: to empower, embolden, and reward behavior I value in myself or others

18. Equality: to treat others as equals, without discrimination; to expect to be treated equitably

19. Excitement: to seek, create, and engage in stimulating or thrilling activities

20. Fairness: to be impartial and just with myself and others

21. Fitness: to maintain or improve my physical and mental health and well-being

22. Flexibility: to adjust and adapt readily to changing circumstances

23. Forgiveness: to be generous in showing grace and reconciliation

24. Freedom: to choose how I live and behave; to help others do the same for themselves

25. Friendliness: to be outgoing, companionable, and agreeable toward others

26. Fun: to be playful, spirited, and light-hearted; to engage in joyful activities

27. Generosity: to be charitable and unselfish; sharing and giving toward myself and others

28. Gratitude: to be thankful; to appreciate aspects of myself, others, and life

29. Honesty: to be truthful and sincere with myself and others

30. Humility: to be humble and modest; to let my achievements speak for themselves

31. Humor: to see and appreciate the witty, comical side of life

32. Impact: to have an effect so what I do is of consequence; to work for what I want, not for what others want from me

33. Independence: to be self-sustaining, self-supportive, and choose my own way of doing things

34. Industry: to be diligent, conscientious, hard-working, and dedicated

35. Intimacy: to open, reveal, and share myself—emotionally and/or physically—in my close personal relationships

36. Justice: to uphold righteousness, honor, and fairness

37. Kindness: to be compassionate, considerate, nurturing, and caring toward myself and others

38. Love: to act affectionately, attentively, and warmly toward myself and others

39. Mindfulness: to be conscious of, open to, and curious about my here- and-now experience

40. Open-mindedness: to be impartial and receptive, see things from the point of view of others

41. Order: to be methodical, meticulous, and organized

42. Patience: to wait calmly and with self-restraint for what I want

43. Persistence: to persevere; to continue resolutely despite problems or difficulties

44. Pleasure: to experience, share, or create enjoyment and delight

45. Power: to strongly influence or wield authority over others; to take charge, lead, command

46. Reciprocity: to build relationships that demonstrate a fair balance of giving and taking

47. Respect: to honor and admire myself and others; be polite, considerate, and hold others in high regard

48. Responsibility: to be accountable for my actions

49. Romance: to display and express love or strong affection

50. Safety: to secure, protect, or ensure my welfare and that of others

51. Self-awareness: to notice my own thoughts, feelings, and actions

52. Self-care: to look after my health and well-being and ensure my needs are met

53. Self-control: to show restraint, self-will, and discipline in accordance with my ideals

54. Self-development: to keep growing, advancing, or improving in knowledge, skills, character, or life experience

55. Sensuality: to create, explore, and enjoy experiences that stimulate the five senses

56. Sexuality: to explore or express desires and passions as they relate to physical urges and drives.

57. Skillfulness: to continually practice and improve my abilities, talents, and gifts; apply myself fully when using them.

58. Soul in the game: to be ethical, have integrity; what I preach and how I live my life are one and the same.

59. Spirituality: to connect with things bigger than and beyond myself

60. Supportiveness: to be helpful, encouraging, and available to myself and others

61. Trust: to be loyal, faithful, dependable, and reliable

62. Insert your own values here.
This activity is adapted from Taylor Pearson's Personal Values in less than 15 minutes.

_____

_____

_____

_____

_____

_____

_____

List your Top 10 values. You may want to combine some and redefine what they encompass.

1. _____

2. _____

3. _____

4. _____

5. _____

6. _____

7. _____

8. _____

9. _____

10. _____

If you get stuck on this activity, ask yourself, "What behavior pushes my buttons the most?" "What drives me crazy?" Maybe it's one of your own behaviors that drives you crazy. You see, when your behavior goes against your values, it will create some inner conflict or physical discomfort. Have you ever experienced that? Write about what comes up for you.

Now it's time to combine and narrow it down to your Top 5 values. Hard, I know, but keep going.

1. _____

2. _____

3. _____

4. _____

5. _____

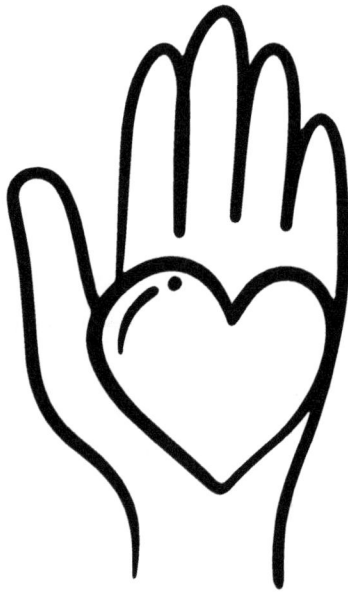

Values Manifesto

Activity

Part of living a mindful life is slowing down enough to be fully present and open to your daily experiences or "moments" so you can act in ways guided by your values.

Take your Top 5 values and create a present tense statement to guide your thinking, feeling, and acting. When you are aligned with your values, regardless of the circumstances that come your way, life is easier to negotiate with less worry and indecision. " I am…"

_____

_____

_____

_____

_____

_____

_____

_____

_____

_____

_____

_____

_____

_____

Mindful Solutions

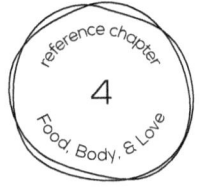

reference chapter

4

Food, Body, & Love

Beginners Mind

Expectancy is allowing the past to direct your future. Beginner's mind is a mindfulness technique that asks you to clear your mind of all past judgments and expectations. Everything is a new experience, all things are possible. Mindfulness is embracing each moment as new; seeing what presents itself in the present moment, without judgment. It's like writing an entirely new script. It involves responding to people, places, and things as if experiencing them for the very first time.

How might things be different if you approached your life this way? Of course, there is a certain amount of wisdom we'd like to bring with us, but the method encourages us not to judge new situations based on what we expect. We are now going to form our opinions based on the new information presented to us. It's a do-over! Share your thoughts about how beginner's mind could decrease your current struggles.

_____

_____

_____

_____

_____

_____

_____

Mindful Solutions

Thought Defusion

Fused Thoughts

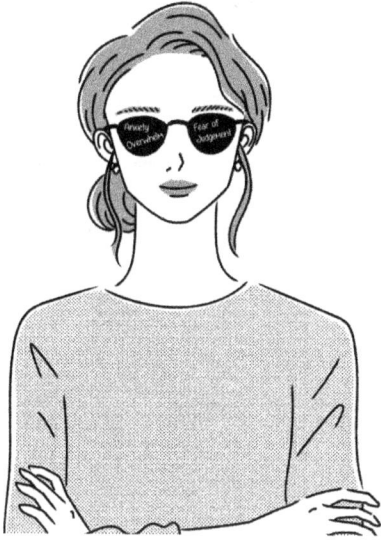

Defused Thoughts

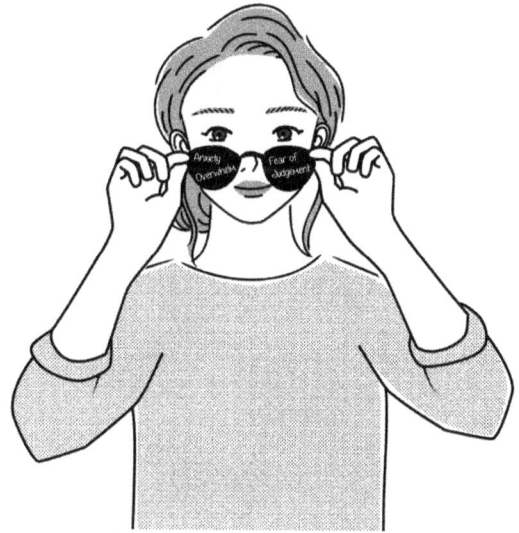

Having fixed, fused thoughts is like wearing glasses that filter everything through the lens of your beliefs. They are so close to you, you don't even see them. You just see squiggly lines comprising your life's landscape.

Defused thoughts allow you to take the lens off to see and decide whether your current beliefs are a good fit for you. Defused thinking gives you the flexibility to choose a different pattern of thought.

Self-inquiry is the willingness to question our core beliefs and things we might consider fact or truths. Self-inquiry diminishes the critical self-talk and assumptions that lead to troublesome emotions and ineffective behaviors.

What are some of your fused thoughts you might want to defuse and shift?

Example: I will always struggle with food and my weight, becomes, I choose to let go of fear and embrace a lifestyle of freedom and care

_____

_____

_____

_____

_____

_____

_____

_____

_____

_____

_____

_____

_____

_____

Self-Care Solution

Unclutter. Create a Sanctuary

Our brain is simple. It gets overwhelmed easily. Contrary to popular productivity theory, multitasking is not effective. I have a "leaky faucet theory" of why we get overwhelmed. Every time we see something that needs to be done or that bothers us, we engage in negative self-talk, "We should be doing more!" and "Why aren't we keeping up?" It's always one more thing. We get overwhelmed and procrastinate, or we shut down altogether. Remember the fear response of collapsing into freeze? That's an extreme example of reacting to it's all too much! Not all personality types react this way, but many of those who struggle with perfectionism do.

An effective self-care solution for keeping your brain clear and body calm is to get organized and minimize distractions. It is important to create surroundings that "spark joy" and foster a twinkle light state of mind.

What could you do to begin uncluttering your life and creating sanctuary spaces of calm? Just one thing: start small. First, take five minutes to come up with a plan of action. Who can you call on to help you? Plenty of people love helping others organize and declutter. Where will you begin?

Plan of Action

8 C's

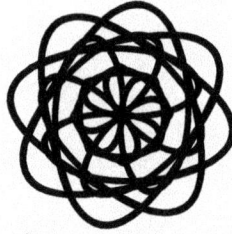

Experience

In this session we will focus on being Clear.

"Be Clear"

Draw a picture, symbol, or create a phrase reminding and anchoring you to the feeling of clarity.

Reflect on things that have brought you clarity in the past. How can you create more clarity in your life?

_____

_____

_____

_____

How can you be clearer in your thinking?

_____

_____

Reflection and Discussion

Reflection: Write freely on insights you've gained from this session.

_____

_____

_____

_____

_____

_____

_____

_____

_____

_____

_____

_____

_____

_____

_____

_____

_____

_____

Discussion: For group leaders:

- Ask if anyone would like to share how their mindset has impacted their life's direction. Validate with compassion.

- Open the group up for a discussion about values and living in accordance with one's values. Allow group members to share their Top 5 values. Expand the conversation to include how changes in thought and behavior could help live a more authentic life.

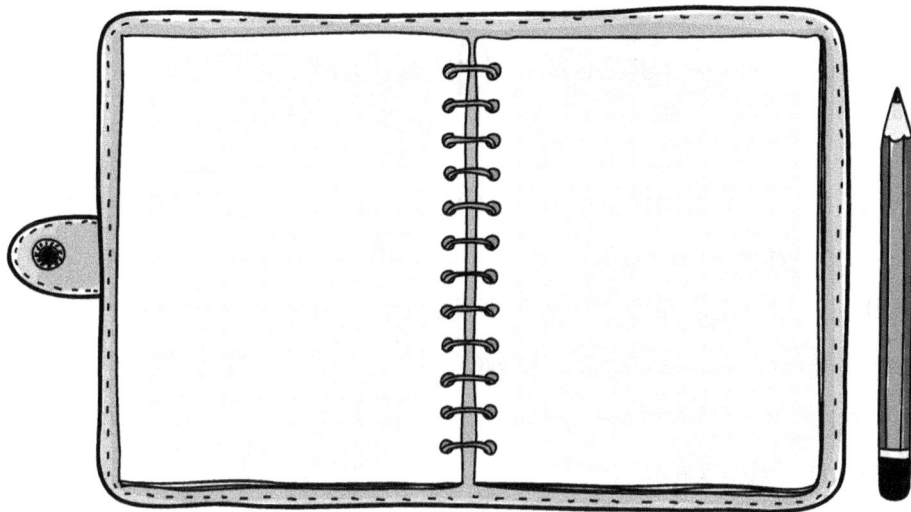

session six

"You will never change your life until you
change something you do daily.
The secret of your success is found in
your daily routine."

John Maxwell

The Habit Connection

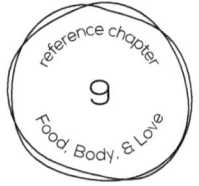

Blame it on your brain. I'm not trying to shirk responsibility here; I'm trying to explain there is no shame in getting caught in the cyclical web of ineffective behavioral habits. Call it addiction, call it disorder, it's a pattern of behavior the brain—computer software of the mind—works hard to keep in place, even though you have good intentions to change it. Change is hard, but it is possible if you understand it means changing the brain. It's not an issue of willpower. It requires compassion and persistence. It also requires strategy.

Habits either support our values or contradict them. Habits tend to be associated with triggers, or stimuli, that activate our thoughts and actions. Triggers can take the form of people, events, circumstances, and even thoughts. Examples include time of day, a physical state or emotion, a person's beliefs, or a place. Being alone used to trigger me to eat even if I wasn't hungry. Being alone meant it was an "opportunity" to eat.

Describe some of your habits.

I have the habit of _____

when _____

I have the habit of _____

when _____

I have the habit of _____

when _____

I have the habit of _____

when _____

I have the habit of _____

when _____

I have the habit of _____

when _____

The Path of Least Resistance

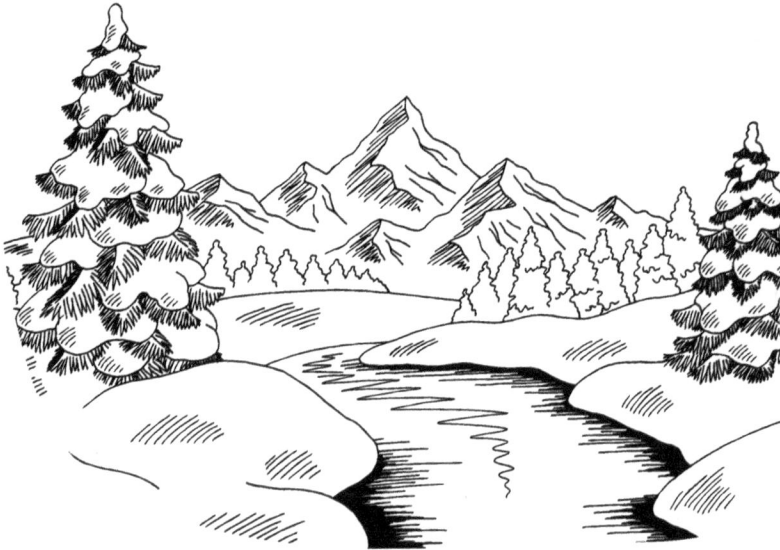

When water from melting snow runs down a mountain, it finds the path of least resistance. Water, with the help of gravity, forms waterfalls, creek beds, and rivers, leading to lakes and oceans. Each year it goes where it has always gone. To divert the water in another direction requires heavy equipment and an engineer. Our brain's neuropathways work much the same way. It takes a heavy dose of mindfulness to elicit the help of our cortex (our thinking brain) to override or redirect a habit. It requires a strategy, which we develop in this session.

Mindfulness is the powerful ability of the human cortex to pause, observe, and choose. It requires energy and a calm (ventral vagal) nervous system. I call it our "bandwidth." If we are stressed and tired, mindfulness can be nearly impossible. Our decisions will be undermined by the sympathetic and dorsal vagal states of our nervous system. When our nervous system is so busy protecting us, there is no energy left to pause and change directions. In essence, unless we can "use our right mind," we are just "our good intentions." We default to our automated habits, the path of least resistance.

This explains why you can have great plans in the morning after a good night's rest yet find yourself doing the same thing you swore you wouldn't do by late afternoon or evening. It is important to have a strategy in place for when you can't think straight, and even for when you still can think straight. It is vital to pay attention to your nervous system throughout the day and use self-care strategies to help you return to the top of the ladder (ventral vagal). If you wait until the end of the day, you may not have the strength to hang on any longer and find you've collapsed at the bottom rung, succumbing to powerful, ingrained habits. Those of you who struggle with attention deficit or who have highly sensitive nervous systems may have to prioritize self-care more than others as a way of life! Self-care is not selfish, it's essential.

Reflect on this lesson. Does your behavior with food make more sense now that you understand the science behind it?

_____

_____

_____

_____

_____

_____

_____

_____

"It's a terrible thing, I think, in life to wait until you're ready.

I have this feeling now that actually no one is ever ready

to do anything. There is almost no such thing as ready.

There is only now."

Hugh Laurie

There are good, protective reasons to procrastinate: perfectionism, fear of failure, or fear of success. Have a conversation with the part of you that defaults to procrastination. Listen to your fearful parts. Validate them. Now revisit your values. Allow your authentic self to speak some truth to your fearful self. Negotiate a willingness to try. Let go of outcome. Outcome is associated with success or failure. Trying is showing up and pivoting in a new direction in this moment.

Share your conversation with your fear part. (Recall your Faces of Fear from "Session Four.")

_____

_____

_____

_____

_____

_____

_____

_____

_____

"You always hold the rights to your effort, but never to your results. Results are entitled to no one. At best, they are on loan and must be renewed each day. All you own is the right to try."

James Clear

Let's discuss the difference between two different types of habits: outcome- vs. identity-based. Outcome-based habits tend to be short term and finite and are based on what you want to achieve. Identity-based habits, on the other hand, focus on who you want to become. Our habits support our identity. We choose to make lifestyle changes to support our values and who we are or want to be. If you want to be an athlete, train like one. If you value self-care or mindfulness, create habits that calm the body and make it feel safe—as described in the self-care solutions found throughout this workbook.

Create a statement of declaration about a new identity in the present tense. Describe habits that will support this new identity. Remember these are not outcome-based habits focused on results, they are identity-based habits focused on who you want to be and how you want to live. Remember, the daily lifestyle habits you choose will support your new identity.

Identity Statement:

_____

_____

Supportive habits:

_____

_____

The Anatomy of a Habit

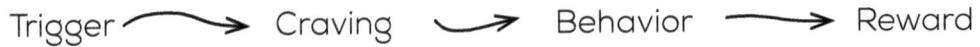

Trigger ⟶ Craving ⟶ Behavior ⟶ Reward

Dopamine is known as the "pleasure" neurotransmitter. It is the neurotransmitter (brain hormone) that makes you feel good after you've eaten food or done anything that activated the brain's reward system.

Dopamine, also responsible for learning new information, is involved in the formation of habits. It compels us, through our cravings and obsessions, to go against our values to obtain the desired reward. Once we obtain that reward, we often realize we didn't need or like it that much after all. Then, never feeling fully satisfied, we try to get more of the reward thinking more will be better. This behavior comes from our primitive survival instincts. If we had not been compelled to seek reward, such as to hunt for food, we would have become extinct. Unfortunately, our brain doesn't shut this survival mechanism down just because we happen to live in an environment of plenty.

There are four stages dopamine goes through in forming a habit. In the process, new neuropathways (brain connections) are formed to keep the habit in place.

Stage One:

Before a habit is learned, dopamine is released the first time you experience the reward. For instance, food.

Stage Two:

Once a trigger is recognized, dopamine begins to rise. This creates a craving.

Stage Three:

Once the habit is learned, dopamine won't rise when a reward is experienced because it already expects it. It just keeps craving.

Stage Four:

If you don't respond to your craving, dopamine will drop, and you will feel out of sorts (crappy). If you return to satisfying your craving, thereby reinforcing the habit, dopamine will spike again as if to say, "I told you not to stop satisfying your craving!" And you thought it was all about willpower.

This is why it is so hard to stop a habit. If it's a positive habit, this is a good thing. If it is a habit that no longer serves you, you will need to diminish it. This will require some brain training! The following is a simple lesson in brain training.

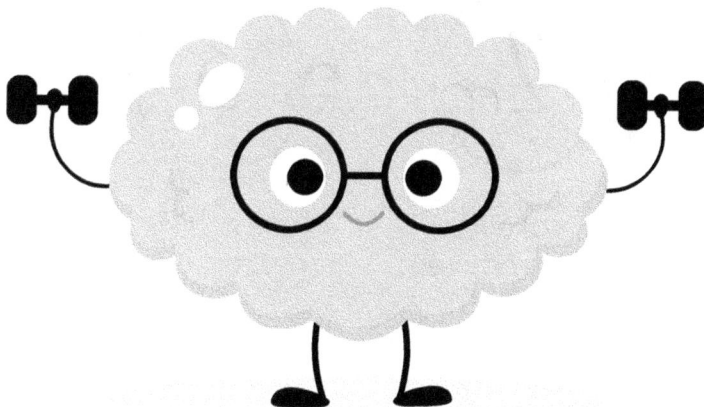

This lesson adapted from James Clear of Atomic Habits

How to Create an Effective Habit

1 Make it Obvious

2 Make it Attractive

3 Make it Easy

4 Make it Satisfying

How to Break an Ineffective Habit

1 Make it Invisible

2 Make it Unattractive

3 Make it Difficult

4 Make it Unsatisfying

Changing Habits

Activity

Diminishing Ineffective Habits

All triggers set off little sequences of thoughts and behaviors that allow you to accomplish attaining your reward. In other words, many mini habits stack on top of one another to create momentum for acquiring your reward. One reward becomes a trigger for another habit.

Let's start by being objective and honest. Ask yourself, what makes it easy for me to get my reward?

Here is an example of a binge habit:

It's six p.m., I'm tired and hungry. I remember my roommate is working late tonight. I start thinking about eating an extra-large pizza all by myself. I pull out my phone and order the pizza on my restaurant app. I take the route home that passes all my favorite fast-food restaurants. Once I pick up the pizza, I notice breadsticks and a liter of cola are on special, so I add them to my order. When driving through the neighborhood, I see a dumpster I can use to dispose of my pizza box, so my roommate won't know I had a binge. Once home, I put on my sweatpants, turn on Netflix, and sit in my easy chair with the pizza on the ottoman. I eat until I am in a state of dissociative bliss. I barely gather myself to dispose of the evidence and get into bed before my roommate arrives home.

There are several triggers in this sequence, how many can you name?

What are the cravings? What are the rewards? Is the pizza the only reward?

_____

_____

_____

What are the mini habits? What thoughts or behaviors make it easier to complete this habit?

_____

_____

_____

In this example, what could you do to make this ineffective habit more invisible, unattractive, difficult, and unsatisfying?

_____

_____

_____

_____

_____

Just thinking about this is probably bringing up fear and anxiety.
That's dopamine at work!

Creating Effective Habits

Using the leaving work scenario established in the last activity, what new behavior(s) could be formed into a new habit?

_____

What positive triggers could be used to make the new habit seem obvious and attractive?

_____

_____

_____

How could you respond to triggers beyond your control to make it easier to maintain your new habit?

_____

_____

What might be the reward for engaging in this new habit? Keep in mind, a reward can be a feeling. What would make the reward satisfying? What reward do you see yourself working toward in this hypothetical scenario?

_____

_____

_____

What behaviors can be put in place to prompt a chain of mini habits that will reinforce one another?

_____

_____

_____

Now it's your turn! Deconstruct one of your ineffective habits and create a new, more effective habit

Share in detail a well-worn habit you would like to diminish.

_____

_____

_____

_____

_____

Identify the triggers involved with this habit.

_____

_____

What is it you are craving? What is the reward you get from satisfying this craving?

_____

_____

What are the mini habits? What thoughts and behaviors keep this habit going?

_____

_____

_____

What new behavior(s) could be formed into a new, more effective habit?

_____

_____

What positive triggers could be used to make the new habit seem obvious and attractive?

_____

_____

What might be the reward for engaging in this new habit? Keep in mind, a reward can be a feeling. What would make the reward satisfying?

_____

_____

_____

What behaviors can be put in place to prompt a chain of mini habits that will reinforce one another?

_____

_____

Values Action Matrix

Activity

Inside (thoughts and feelings)

Away from values

Toward values

Outside (behaviors and actions)

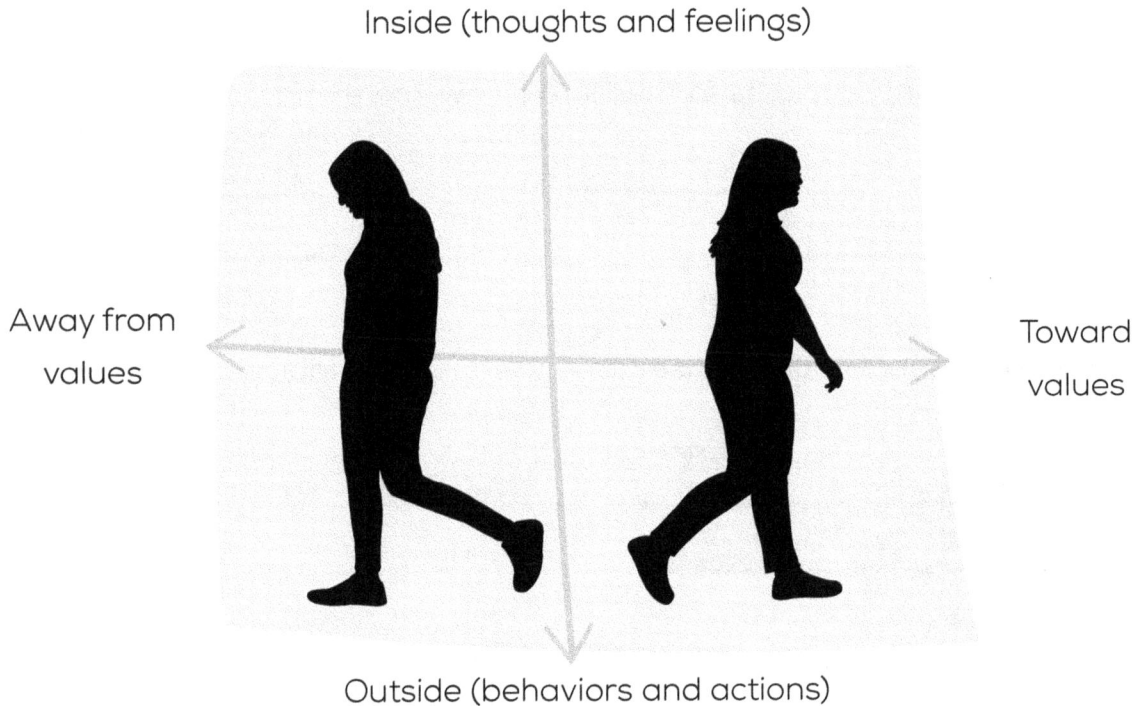

In the matrix above, there are four quadrants of influence that govern our decision-making process. Our thoughts and feelings (internal factors) are depicted in the top half of the matrix. Our behaviors and actions (external factors) are depicted in the bottom half. The right and left sides of the matrix are divided by whether we pivot toward our values or away from them. We are faced with thousands of choices every day. As you can see, the choices we make are determined by our thoughts, feelings, behaviors, actions, and our commitment to our values.

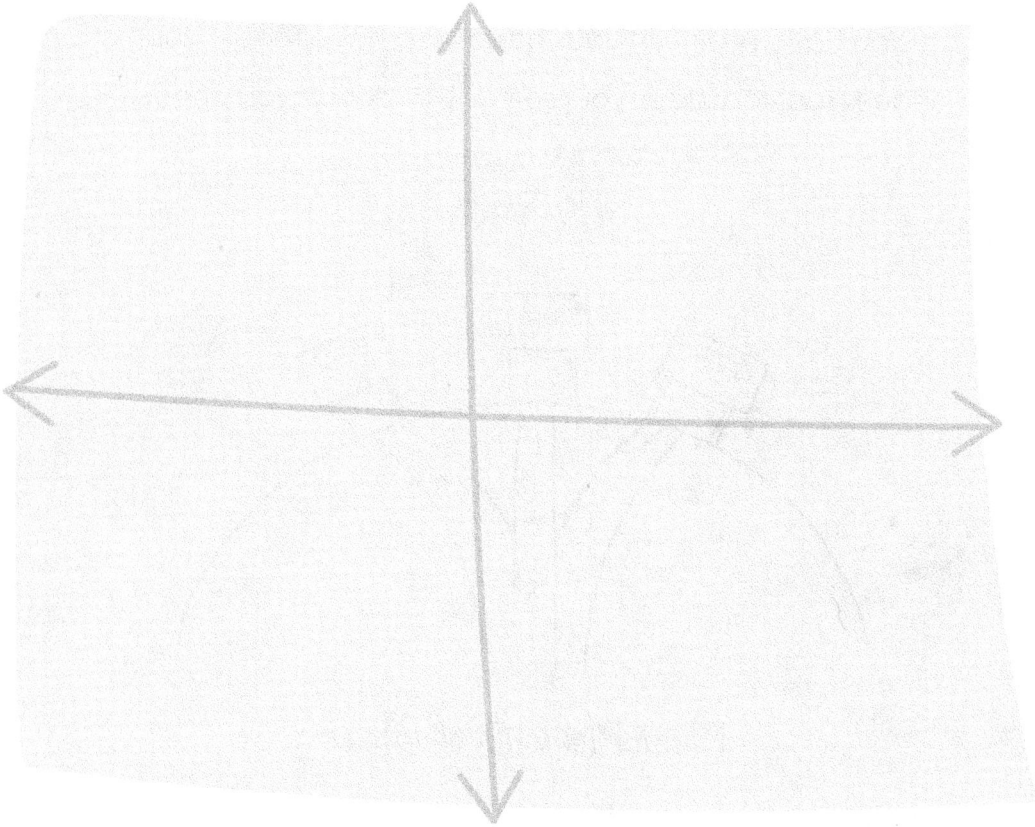

Let's work through the quadrants.

- In the upper left-hand quadrant, list the thoughts and feelings that tend to influence you away from your valued direction.

- In the lower left-hand quadrant, list behaviors and actions that tend to move you away from your valued direction.

- In the upper right-hand quadrant, list the thoughts and feelings that tend to influence you toward your valued direction.

- In the lower right-hand quadrant, list behaviors and actions that move you toward your valued direction.

This activity is adapted from Stephen Hays' ACT therapy.

"You have brains in your head. You have feet in your shoes. You can steer yourself any direction you choose."

Dr. Seuss

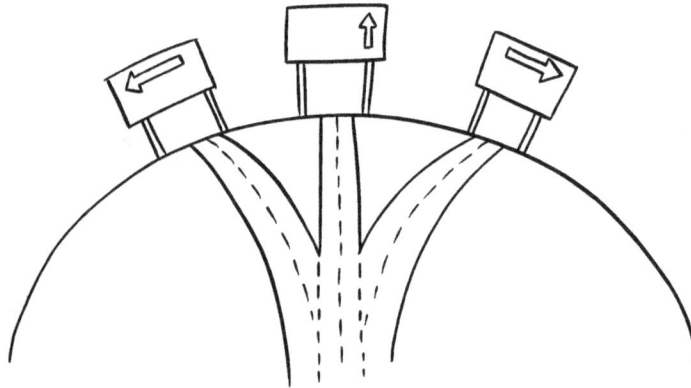

Micro Moments of Choice

We can have all the insight and plans in the world, but if we do not act, nothing will change. Often, we are frozen in a state of inaction. We feel stuck. We have discussed how perfectionism, the fear of outcomes beyond our control, and fear of making a wrong decision can convince us that staying where we are is safer than changing.

I have introduced identity-based habits as small pivots in the direction of your values. The accumulation of these small pivots, over time, will create new outcomes and results in your life.

Each moment provides an opportunity to pivot toward your valued direction. You can start out having a bad day, but the mindset you choose can help turn it into a good day. You can start over in any moment. You do not have to wait until New Year's Day, Monday, or your birthday. You can make a different decision right now. That is empowering!

Away from my Valued Direction   *Valued Direction*

If you turn toward your valued direction more often than away from it, you will move closer to a life of value and meaning. The example above illustrates how your cumulative decisions can change the course of your day, and ultimately your life.

Mindful Solutions

Speed Bumps and Guardrails.

Speed bumps slow you down, force you to pause, and interrupt the trajectory of your mindless automated habit. Have you ever driven the same route so many times you can't even remember how you got from point A to point B? This is what I am talking about! It's time to wake yourself up!

List all the speed bumps that could slow down or interrupt a mindless eating habit.

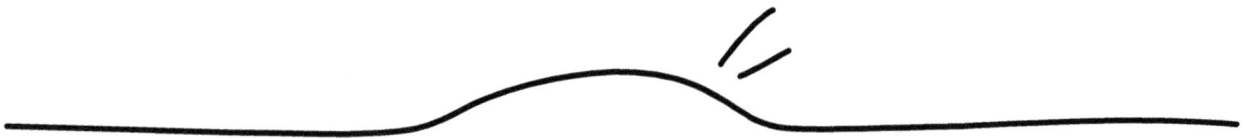

_____

_____

_____

_____

_____

_____

Guardrails keep you from straying off your new intended pathway or habit. They provide the structure needed to keep you on track. Remember, it is important to create strategies for when you can't think straight as well as for times when you can.

What guardrails can you put in place before you are too tired and stressed to resist temptation? Remember to make it easy. Anything requiring significant brain power will not be included as part of the solution. Trust me, from experience, you won't do anything hard.

List all the guardrails you can think of to help keep you on track with your new habit.

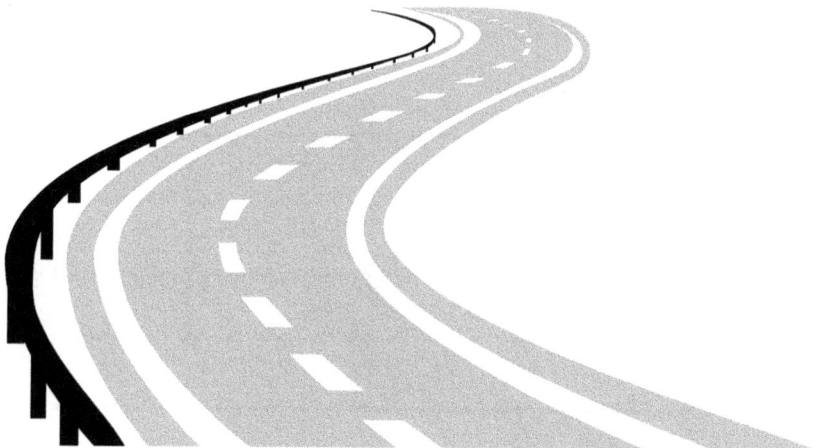

solution

8 C's

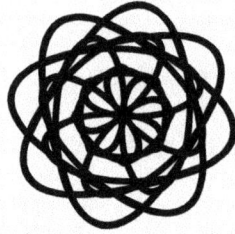

Experience

In this session we will focus on Creativity.

"Be Creative"

As you step out of fear and allow creativity to flow, ideas blossom and allow you to produce beautiful, imaginative things. Draw or write something to remind you to express your creativity.

How have you expressed your creativity in the past?

_____

_____

What have you created lately?

_____

_____

What are things you dream about creating, yet haven't pursued or completed?

_____

_____

Reflection and Discussion

Reflection: Use this space to write freely about any insights gained from this chapter, or anything you choose to commit to as you move in the direction of your values.

Discussion and Activities for Group Leaders

- Ask if anyone, or all, would care to share their reflections on this chapter.

- Ask the group if anyone would care to share the discussion between their fear parts and authentic self when releasing habits that no longer serve them.

- Discuss the Speed bumps and Guardrails activity. Have the group brainstorm ideas for implementing speed bumps and guardrails to help diminish ineffective habits and create more effective ones.

- Discuss the Values Action Matrix Activity. Have the group share the contents of their quadrants. Are there commonalities among the group?

- Discuss the concept of hope. Do they believe change is possible? Why or why not?

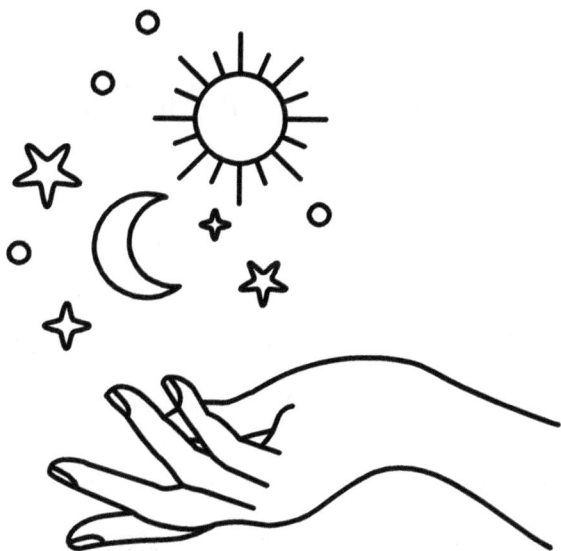

session seven

"You don't have a soul. You *are* a soul.
You *have* a body."

C.S. Lewis

Do These Boobs Make Me Look Fat?

reference chapter
7
Food, Body, & Love

The relationship you have with your body is the most constant and enduring relationship you will ever have in your life. You are together from the beginning until you part at death. The image you have of your body is influenced by the experience of living in it... and the reactions of others to it.

Whether you share this activity with others or not, it is important to speak your truth about what it is like to live in your body. How do you experience it today?

_____

_____

_____

_____

_____

_____

_____

_____

_____

_____

_____

_____

_____

You have a subjective mental image of your own body. This image is established through self-observation and noting the reactions of others. It tends to be an extrinsic measure of physical appearance, but it can also be influenced by our interoceptive or "felt" internal sensations, along with our comparisons and expectations.

Our body image is greatly affected by the culture we live in and the norms and biases of our media, medical system, families, and peers.

What influences or experiences have shaped your image of your body? What biases have you endured? Who made your body their business?

Hello Body, I've Missed You.

Activity

How do we begin to heal our relationship with our body? It starts with mindset.

You don't have to hate your body, but you don't have to love it either. Take a neutral stance toward it. It's not about liking how it looks, it's about coexisting in collaboration with it. You depend on your body to move, think, and exist. If your body isn't well, you don't feel well. Your body determines your opportunities in life, so don't let a poor relationship with it limit your life or create a small existence.

How do we befriend our body? How do we reconcile with it and start anew?

Begin a dialogue with your body in the form of a letter. Start with, "Hello."

Hello, Body,

_____

_____

_____

_____

_____

_____

_____

_____

_____

If your body could speak, what would it say to you? Allow it to tell you what it needs to restore the relationship and move forward.

Dear _____,

_____

_____

_____

_____

_____

_____

_____

_____

_____

_____

_____

_____

_____

_____

_____

_____

_____

_____

Some helpful hints for changing how you feel about your body.

- Stay neutral and nonjudgmental. Accept it exactly as it is in the moment.

- Focus on function and utility. When did we decide to enter it into a beauty pageant?

- Focus on what you appreciate about it; ignore the things that bother you.

- Stop checking and comparing. Skip activities that promote checking and comparing.

- Move more. Moving your body for thirty minutes can change your experience of it.

- Focus on your "felt" experience rather than sight evaluation. Look for and engage in things that give you more energy, clarity of thought, and strength.

- Reclaim it from anyone who thought it was their business discussing it in the first place.

- Let go of expectations regarding its size. Treat it well, engage in self-care, make it feel safe. The size of your body is its business. If it wants to be a different size, it will decide.

- Get rid of anything that makes you feel like your body isn't right or good enough. Get rid of clothes that don't fit, remove a mirror if you need to, dump the scale. Ask others to stop talking about it.

- Challenge media images and photoshop technology used to manipulate reality.

- Add some of your own...

_____

_____

_____

_____

_____

_____

_____

_____

_____

_____

Movement Does a Body Good

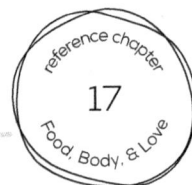

Activity

Exercise is a dirty word for some. It has become connected to calories and prescriptive formulas of "no pain, no gain." We either become compulsive about it or resistant to it. It seems our relationship with exercise also needs some healing. We need to put joy back into moving our bodies.

The human body was designed to move. Exercise is not only good for your body, but also for your brain. Exercise helps with learning, attention, and your mood. It is "brain fertilizer." The body loves exercise! Here are some reasons why:

- Improves sleep
- Reduces pain
- Increases strength and balance
- Improves immunity
- Stimulates digestion
- Improves blood sugar metabolism
- Increases energy
- Decreases anxiety
- And, yes, it tones the vagus nerve!

If your eyes are rolling right about now, and your rebellious parts are pushing back on the subliminal "you should exercise" message, take a breath. Let's start from the beginning and approach this from a unique perspective.

To begin, try to shift your mindset about exercise. Approach it as a self-care practice. It's not about fighting with the body but helping it heal and feel better physically and emotionally. Start small. Implement the five-minute rule, meaning, you can do *anything* for five minutes. Challenge old beliefs. Find safe places to work out. Wear comfortable clothes. Try something fun, or pair exercising with someplace, something, or someone you enjoy.

Activities	paired with	Things I Enjoy
Spending time with a friend		*Walking*

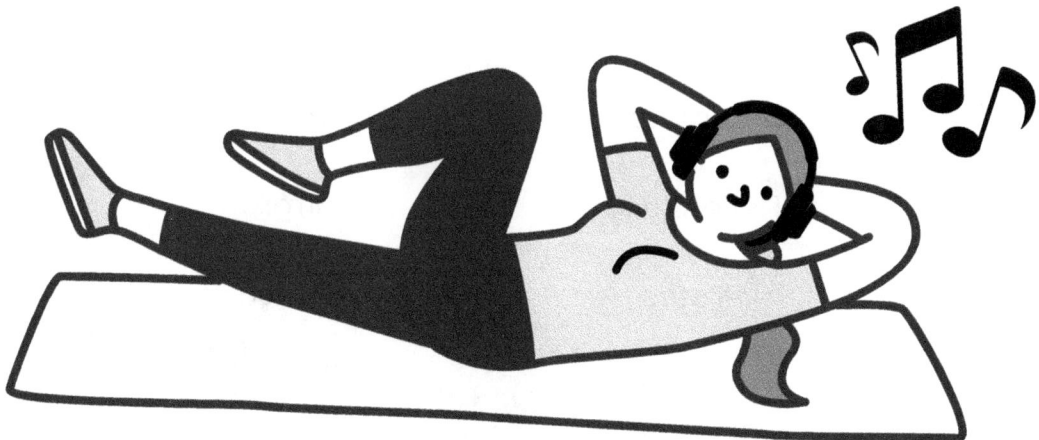

Self-Care Solutions

Embodied Practices

What is an embodied practice? Calming the body and toning the vagal nerve are healing for the body and mind. Any practice that connects you to the sensations and felt experience of your body is embodied. It is especially important for those who have detached from their bodies from the neck down years ago, or have declared war with their body in a constant struggle. You can use sensations of our body as a tool to develop awareness, presence, to self-regulate our nervous system, feel whole, find balance, feel connected, know ourselves and be empowered.

What are embodied practices?

Yoga	Heat Therapy
Tai Chi	Acupuncture
Qigong	Stretching Breathwork
Massage	Cryotherapy
Joint Compression	Hydrotherapy
Reflexology	Infrared
Pilates	Other...

Do you have any experience with these practices? Describe. Are you curious about trying any of them? Why or why not?

_____

_____

_____

_____

_____

_____

_____

_____

solution

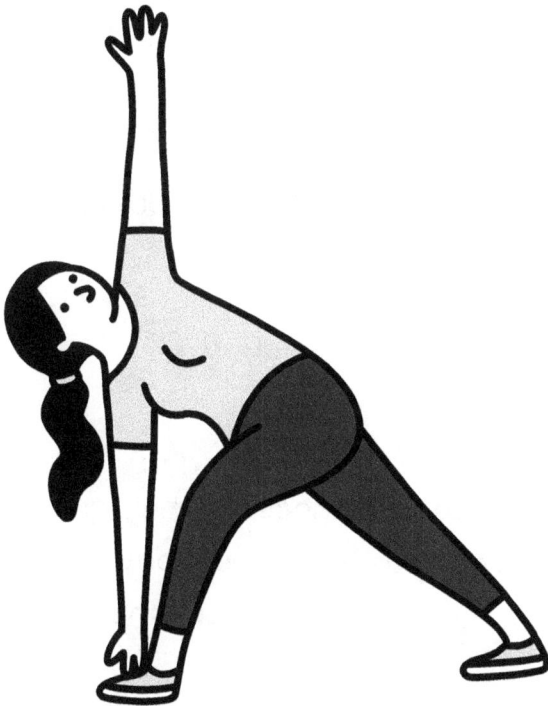
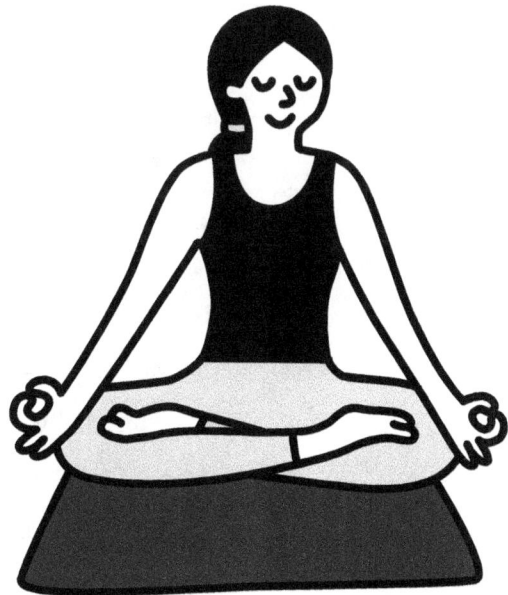

Self-Care Solutions

Play/Sport/Dance

We have learned about the sympathetic nervous system's fight or flight response when danger is evident or perceived. We have also learned about the ventral vagal state characterized by feeling safe, calm, and connected. I am going to introduce a hybrid state activated during movement.

Exercise, done in the spirit of play, sport, and dance, activates the sympathetic nervous system via increased heart and lung activity but does so in the absence of fear. Exercise you hate is not health promoting because it elicits a fear or anxiety response. (I'm thinking elementary school dodge ball. Eek!) Exercise you enjoy combines the activation of the sympathetic nervous system with the ventral vagal state, especially if you are having fun. You are sympathetically aroused—heart rate is up, breathing is accelerated, blood is diverted to your muscles while feeling safe, connected, and having a great time. What a win-win! Mental and physical health are supported at the same time!

When we play, engage in sports, or dance together, we are co-regulating:

- Reciprocity—engaging in pleasant mutual exchange
- Movement without inhibition—you're not worried about what you look like
- Face to face interactions—we are social beings!
- Proximity—being physically close to others; connecting through touch
- The use of music or rhythm—connecting us to internal body rhythms
- Vocalizations: singing or humming—great for stimulating the vagus nerve

In these moments, there is a synergy taking place that brings our spirit alive. Most of these special moments occur while being with others. No wonder I love pickleball, cycling, Peloton classes.

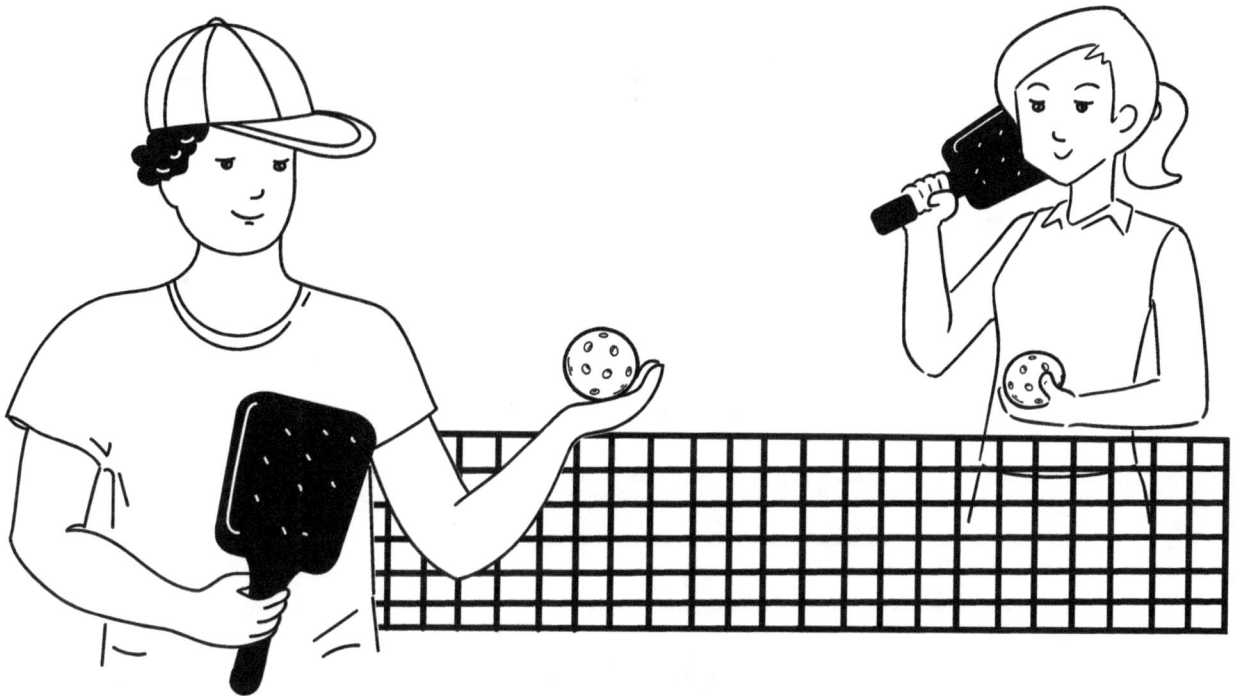

Reflect on the Activity-Pairing assignment.

How many involved these co-regulatory factors: sympathetic + ventral vagal?

_____

_____

_____

_____

_____

_____

_____

_____

_____

_____

_____

_____

_____

_____

Self-Care Solutions

Music and Rhythm

Working with our natural rhythms is vital to healing from trauma. Music and rhythm have been used in all cultures for centuries to calm anxious nervous systems. Our bodies love sound and movement because it indicates safety and continuity. As a baby in the womb, the beating heart and rocking body movements of our mother created a baseline for comfort.

Rhythm can regulate the body in various ways:

- Using gentle, rhythmic breathing to slow a rapid heart rate when stressed is the most basic and reliable. It is also always available.
- Being outdoors resets our body to the circadian rhythm of the sun and the seasons.
- The rhythm of routine reassures us of the constants in our life. I once heard, "The brain loves novelty, but the body rests in routine." Wise words.
- The rhythm of movement also calms the body. Rocking chairs, playground swings, and hammocks are good examples.
- Big exercise balls are good for sitting on and rocking back and forth.
- Use of a "rebounder" or mini trampoline. The jumping rhythm soothes the nervous system and circulates lymphatic fluids.
- Our ear drums are a portal to the vagus nerve. Frequency and vibration stimulate the nervous system and tone the vagus nerve to help us feel calm and safe.
- Singing, chanting, and humming, as previously mentioned. Also, drumming circles, singing bowls, and tuning forks are used worldwide to regulate the nervous system.

- Any music you love can be helpful, but music played or recorded at sixty to eighty beats per minute is especially soothing—like the beating of our heart.

As a polyvagal therapist, I have been trained in a special form of music therapy called Safe and Sound Protocol. Many of my clients have participated in this form of therapy and benefited greatly.

List activities you perform regularly, or are curious about starting, that can ground your body to a sense of safety. How might music and rhythm be a healer in your life?

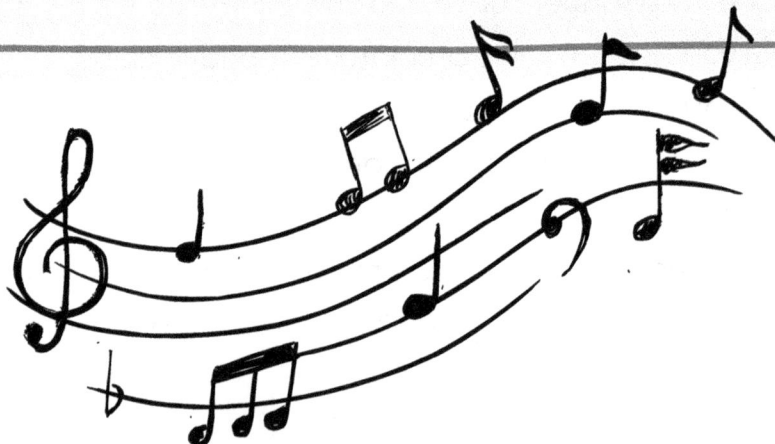

8 C's

Experience

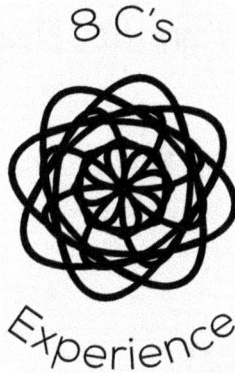

In this session we will focus on Confidence.

"Be Confident"

Draw a picture, symbol or phrase reminding and anchoring you to the feeling of confidence.

Reflect and list things that brought you confidence in the past.

_____

_____

_____

_____

What can you insert into your daily routine to spark your confidence?

_____

_____

_____

Reflection and Discussion

Reflection: Use this space to write freely about any insights gained from this chapter.

_____

_____

_____

_____

_____

_____

_____

_____

_____

_____

_____

_____

_____

_____

_____

_____

_____

_____

_____

Discussion and Activities for Group Leaders

- Ask if anyone would like to share their experience of living in their body and/or influences contributing to their body image. Tend to feelings.

- Ask if anyone is willing to share their letters to and from their body. This is an extremely vulnerable assignment, yet, when spoken out loud can be empowering and helpful to self and others in the group.

- Lead the group in brainstorming ideas for improving one's body image.

- Discuss the paradigm shift needed to go from seeing exercise as punishment to embracing movement as a healer. Allow participants to share their ideas for using movement to heal and care for their bodies.

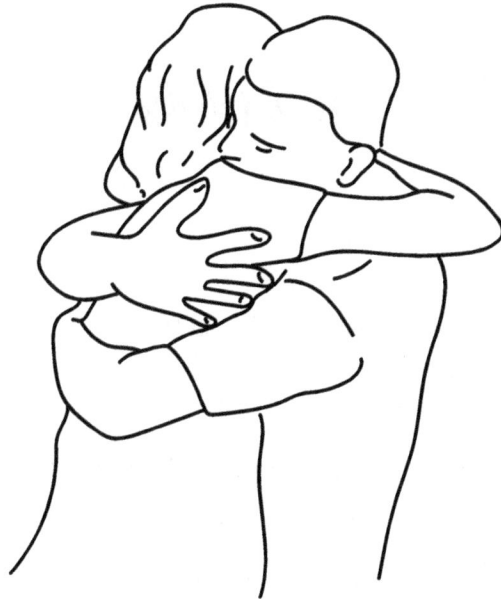

session eight

"God is the designer of successful
relationships, Love and kindness draw
us in, not fear and intimidation."

Dr. Kari Anderson

Love Heals

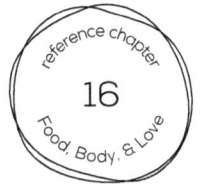

Our bodies thrive in a state of love.

We are hardwired for connection; it's a biological imperative. Our health and happiness depend on it.

When studying the neurobiology of love and bonding, our vagus nerve along with neuropeptides—hormones—respond to love and fear. Their interaction explains how our body influences emotion, attachment, and communication. When love predominates, we find ourselves in the parasympathetic nervous system state known as ventral vagal. In this state, we are "without fear" and feel safe and free to connect with others.

Individuals who access this physiological state often can easily default to altruism, compassion, gratitude, and happiness. These individuals are often described as warm and tender-hearted, and they have a higher resilience to stress. They also have higher levels of oxytocin—the love hormone—and lower levels of cortisol—the stress hormone. This distribution of hormones keeps their level of systemic inflammation low, correlating to good mental and physical health. They have a "chill" personality and can calm down easily when upset. They have a sharper memory and can tap into a clear, creative mindset. No wonder the ventral vagal state is considered our most authentically human state!

Fear and Relationships

We live in a world of mistrust, competition, and divisiveness. Why are relationships so difficult? In a word: fear. Rather than form bonds of connection, we adopt patterns of protection. We don't often recognize our behavior as fear based. We get used to living in a chronic fight or flight response. It becomes "normal" to live in state of sympathetic nervous system activation. It's a state of high alert, ever ready for action and mobilization. When stressed, people either respond with fight behaviors or flight behaviors. Modern day stressors may not evoke beating a wild beast with a tree limb or running for the nearest cave, but our nervous system still reacts the same. We go into protection and survival mode.

Today's fight behaviors tend to be expressed as violent outbursts, chronic anger, defensiveness, criticizing, arguing, and yelling. It can manifest as strategies of control or manipulation or mean-spiritedness, jealousy, or rebellion.

Flight behaviors tend to be expressed as avoiding, stonewalling, disconnecting, and turning away. These behaviors may lead to false attachments or love substitutes, such as food, substances, love and sex addictions, gambling, or overwork. In other words, the person leaves the fearful situation behind by finding something or someone else to soothe or distract them.

According to polyvagal theory, when these behaviors no longer protect us from chronic fear, we enter a third state called the dorsal vagal response. It's a frozen state of hiding, withdrawing, shutting down, and dissociating, as if the individual is unconsciously feigning death. Their focus narrows. They become depressed and live in a toxic state of shame. They feel beaten down, unloved, and unlovable. In some cases, people in the dorsal vagal state die of real or perceived loneliness.

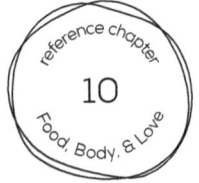

Signals of Fear and Safety

We have an abundant network of nerves located in our face and heart area, making up what is called the *social engagement system.* We unconsciously scan our environment looking for cues to let us know when it's safe to proceed.

You can think of the three branches of the autonomic nervous system like a human traffic light. The ventral vagal state is the green light, giving the "go ahead and live your best life" signal. When in danger, the yellow light sends out a warning to protect us through fight or flight. If our body senses a death threat, it collapses into the red-light state of stop, drop, and play dead.

Since we are wired for connection, the green light usually dominates. Unfortunately, many of us have been rewired by our life experiences. Now we have a heightened sense of danger and tend to default to a pattern of protection. This is especially true if we have endured trauma along the way. Most don't identify themselves as victims of trauma, but trauma is a wound, and many of us bring relational wounds from the past into our current relationships. It takes time to identify our "raw spots" and what triggers us to maintain the well-worn patterns of protection.

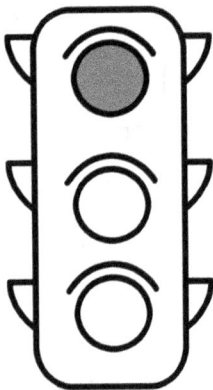

Green
Ventral Vagal

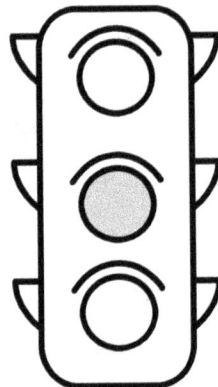

Yellow
Sympathetic

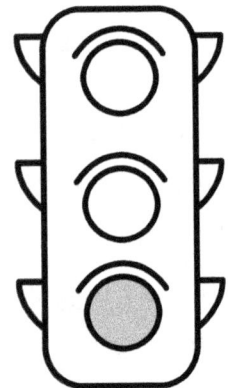

Red
Dorsal Vagal

When we are surrounded by safe people in a safe environment, our nervous system gives us the green light to engage with others face-to-face. We allow eye contact, facial expression, vocalizations, and gestures to support coregulation of our autonomic nervous system. The "gazing effect," or face-heart-connection, takes place when our bodies feel safe with one another. It allows for the intimacy of "being seen and known." Oxytocin is released as we touch, talk, and laugh, creating more opportunities for engaging and bonding.

Our mind and body function best in this state of engagement. To be human is to link heart and face. Our heart rhythms literally begin to align.

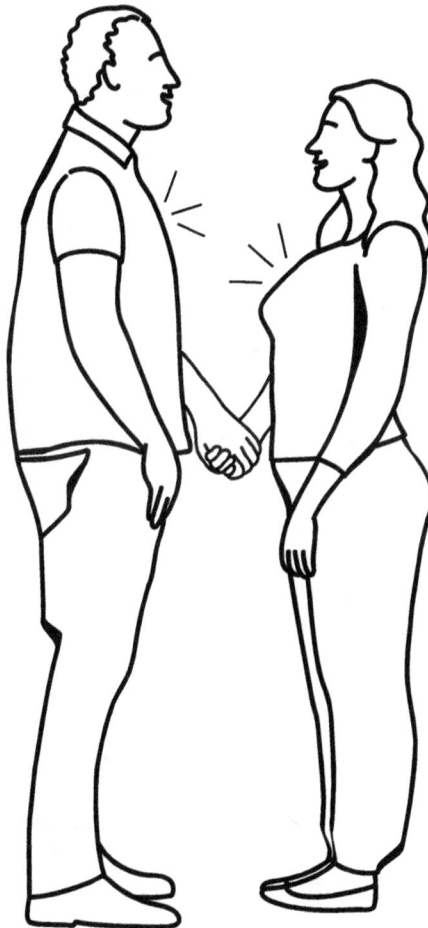

Moving Toward Safer Relationships

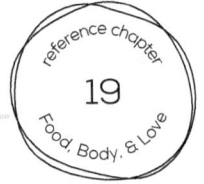

reference chapter
19
Food, Body, & Love

Activity

Start with a relationship inventory.

List people you feel free to be yourself with. We usually feel better after spending time with them.

_____

_____

_____

_____

_____

_____

List people you feel uneasy to share your thoughts and feelings with. You tend to feel worse about yourself after having spent time with them.

_____

_____

_____

_____

_____

_____

When possible, we want to create healthy boundaries. These allow us to spend more time with safe people in our lives and limit time spent with those who make us uneasy. Unhealthy friendships and workplace interactions are easier to change than relationships bonded by marriage or blood.

Setting boundaries with those closest to us can create conflict and hard feelings. Be gentle, seek guidance from a marriage and family therapist, and remember we do not have to end relationships to create more safety in them. The exception is if you are in a dangerous or abusive situation. In that instance, reach out to a local domestic violence hotline.

What are some healthy boundaries you could put in place?

Neuroception and Relationships

Our bodies respond biologically to rudeness. They react on a cellular level to acts of dismissal. If we bid for our partner's attention or support and get no response, it can ignite a strong feeling of rejection that hits us in the gut. In fact, the expressionless face of a mother in response to her baby's cries for love and attention can render the baby inconsolable.

Why is the fear of rejection so primal? Being left out or kicked out of the clan could be life threatening to humans. It elicits fear and panic because we need others to survive. We also crave others turning toward us with respect and admiration, implicitly communicating, "I value you."

To create a safe, approachable environment for intimacy, soften the muscles around your eyes, lean in, tilt your head with interest, and use a singsong tone in your voice. Good parents and good pet owners understand this concept! Once safety is established, through coregulation and touch, which releases oxytocin, individuals allows themselves enough vulnerability to fall easily into the arms of another.

A True Partnership

As adults, we often forget the niceties, expecting our partners to "just get over it." We may label them as "too sensitive," forgetful—or never knowing—about their hardwired physiological states. This vulnerability needs to be accepted and respected. Love needs to be approached with an open hand, freely given and received... never forced.

Fear prompts some of us to control and manipulate, sending others running for fear of being trapped. One partner will yell, the other retreats, prompting the first to run after the second, further frightening them. It becomes a protective cycle of fight and flight where angry faces and loud tones contribute to a no-win situation.

When a couple is in conflict, it is vital to give each other some time and space to calm down. If they remain in a sympathetic state of fear, behavioral patterns of protection only heighten. In a true partnership, each partner needs to help the other feel safe before proceeding with difficult conversations. Learning each other's triggers and habitual responses helps identify the blocks to safe communication. It's not about blaming, but rather teaching each other what helps or hurts when creating safety. Finding a spirit of gratitude, fondness, and compassion cultivates mutual sensitivity.

This all starts with you. Waiting for your partner to change is a form of avoidance. Navigating the complexities of a successful relationship is easier if you understand your own nervous system states. Try to stay curious and take on the role of a scientist when learning about your nervous system responses. Discover how to notice, interpret, and explain your nervous states without judgment. Understand your triggers and your well-developed patterns of protection. Befriend the nervous system, as it is instinctively your protector. Healing begins with awareness.

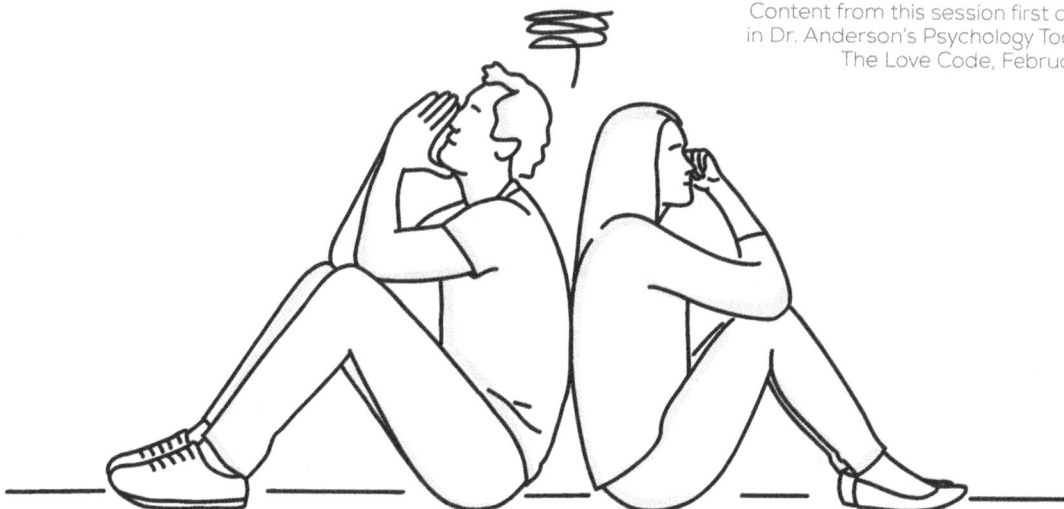

Content from this session first appeared in Dr. Anderson's Psychology Today Blog, The Love Code, February 2021.

Understanding your own patterns of protection.

What do you do when your partner yells or gets loud?

_____

_____

What happens when you "bid" for attention and it is not reciprocated?

_____

_____

Do you tend to pick fights or flee from them? What about your partner?

_____

_____

What do you notice about your nervous system states that may be affecting your relationships?

_____

_____

_____

_____

_____

_____

What do you need to feel safe in your relationships with others?

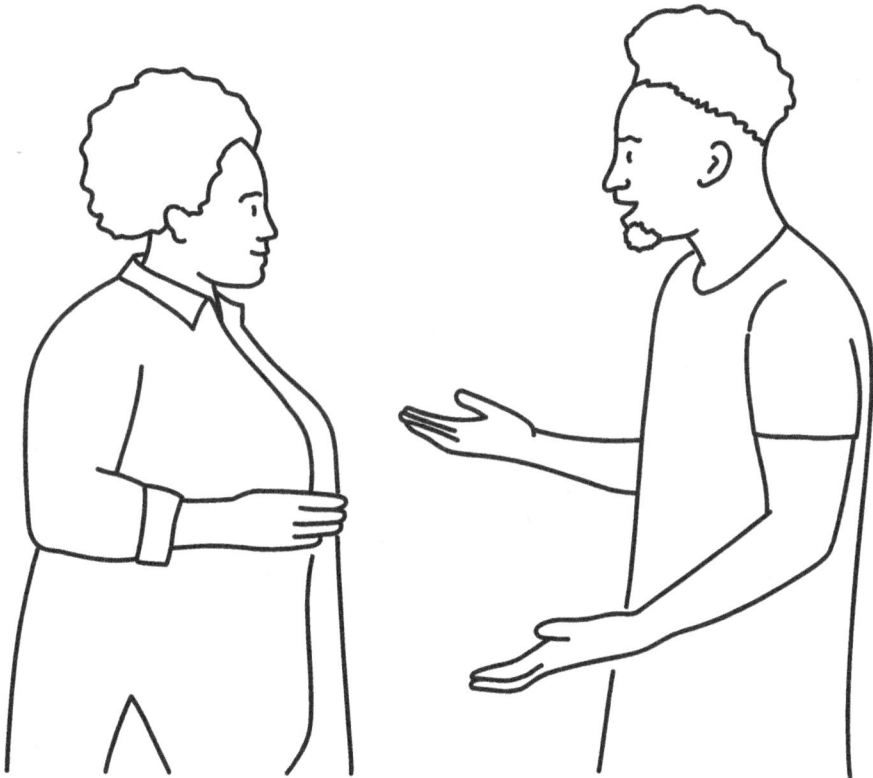

_____

_____

_____

_____

_____

_____

_____

Back to Love Basics

Activity

Some of us don't feel safe in relationships anymore. You may have withdrawn, made a habit of isolating yourself, or avoid opportunities to socialize. Body image combined with post-COVID anxieties may be contributing to your situation.

It is not uncommon for those who have depended on food as their primary nervous system regulator and relational attachment to have difficulty transitioning back to others for support. It is especially hard when one has been beaten down by micro-aggressions due to social biases and unsafe environments. Healing can be a slow journey. Be compassionate with yourself, but start trying to break out of ineffective habits of isolation.

Start by visualizing safe people and noticing how your body reacts:

_____

Visualize unsafe people and notice how your body reacts:

_____

Identify safety cues you get from those you feel safe with. Describe.

_____

Identify danger cues you get from those you find unsafe. Describe.

_____

Practice touch. Start with yourself, hand on heart. Describe.

_____
_____

Try Massage. Start by applying lotion to yourself. Once that is comfortable, move on to a professional massage. Describe.

_____
_____
_____

Practice hugs. Start by giving yourself a big bear hug. Move on to allowing hugs from others, hold long enough for oxytocin to surge. Describe.

_____
_____
_____
_____

Engage in play and laughter with others. Describe.

_____
_____
_____
_____

Practice face- to- face communication. Describe.

_____

_____

_____

_____

_____

Practice eating with others face- to- face. Describe.

_____

_____

_____

_____

_____

Practice setting boundaries with others. Describe.

_____

_____

_____

_____

_____

Hearts Aligned

The Healing Presence of Pets.

There is something special about the love we feel toward our pets and the authenticity of the love we receive from them in return. There is a "Pedigree® Hearts Aligned" video that tracks love bonds formed between humans and dogs by measuring heart rate variability or HRV. (Recall, HRV is the amount of time between heartbeats. More time between beats means increased variability and a greater degree of resilience and wellbeing.) When owners and dogs are apart, they are largely dysregulated and have faster heart rates. Within minutes of being reunited, their heart rates begin to align in rate and rhythm. Amazing! This is coregulation at its finest. It occurs through the heart-face connection, or social engagement system, of the body.

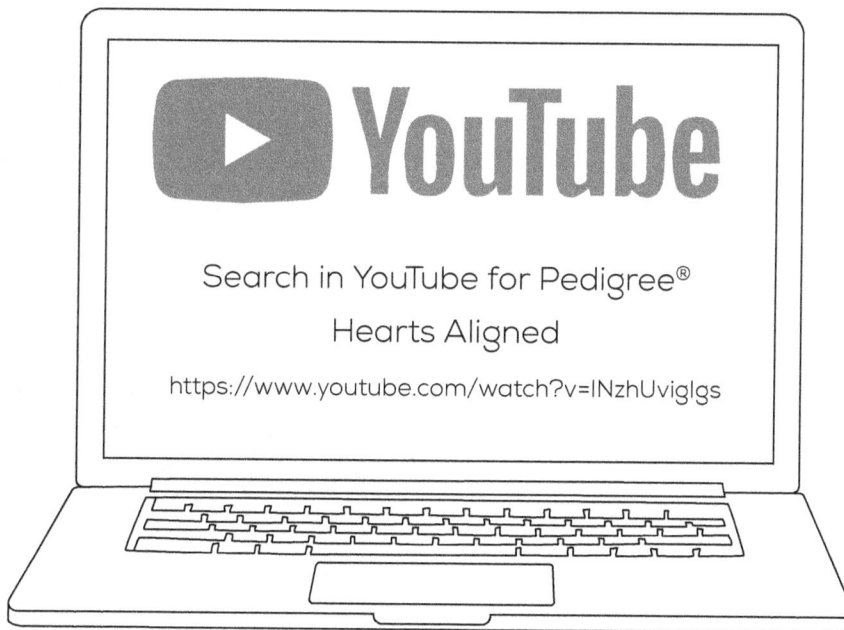

Search in YouTube for Pedigree®
Hearts Aligned

https://www.youtube.com/watch?v=lNzhUviglgs

After watching the video, reflect on your feelings.

_____

_____

_____

_____

_____

Do you have a pet? Have you ever had a pet with this close of a bond?

_____

_____

_____

_____

_____

People with pets live longer and healthier lives. Our pets are nervous system regulators!

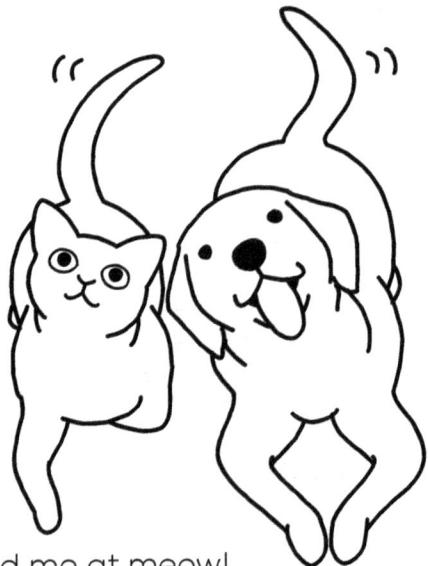

You had me at meow!

Mindful Solutions

"The Scientist"

If you tend to take on others' feelings and emotions, find you take things personally, and are often upset by other people's actions, consider becoming a scientist.

This involves the act of observing others through a curious lens. Collect data with the understanding that the "subject's thoughts, feelings, and actions have nothing to do with you as a researcher. Allow for an imaginary space or force field, perhaps a one-way window between you and those you are observing. A good scientist will also use a Beginner's Mind to prevent examiner bias. Hmm, very interesting.

Experiment with a subject and detail your scientific notes.

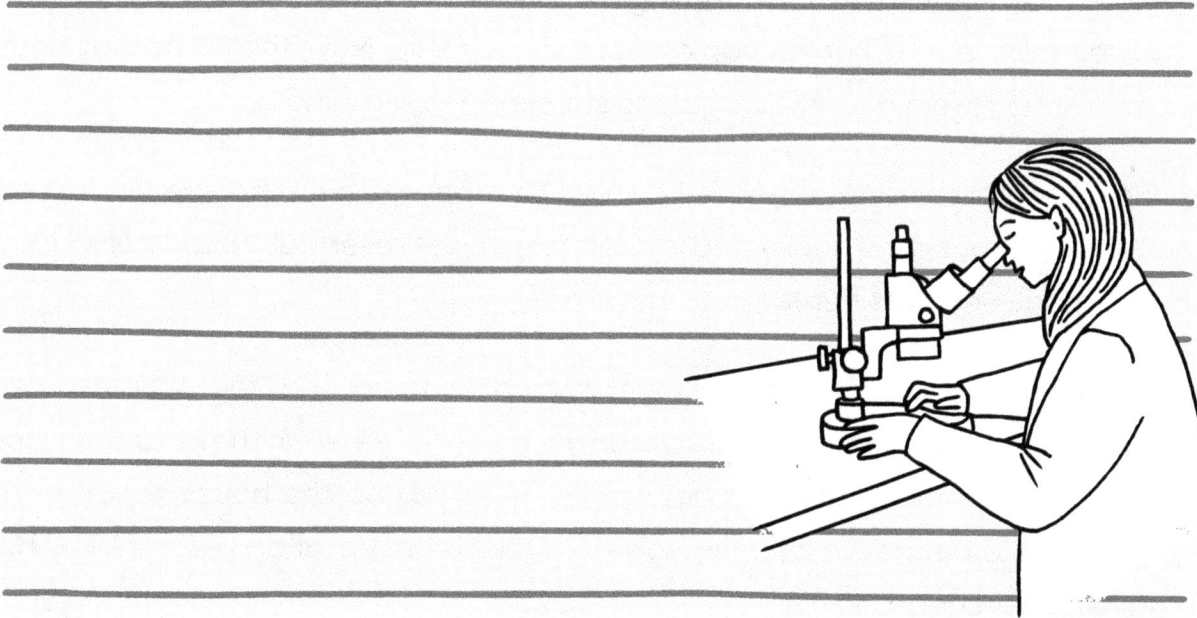

Self-Care Solution

Communicating Your Needs with Assertive Scripts

"I have been thinking..."

"I have been feeling... or I felt..."

"What I need is"...

"One thing that might help is..."

It is important to communicate your needs as something you require, desire, or deserve rather than something you want someone to do. Believe it or not, there are many ways to meet your needs. We often get fixated on what we think needs to happen, rather than getting to the source of the deeper, true need.

For instance, many of my younger female clients come to me lamenting they need a boyfriend (or girlfriend). In searching for the root of the need, it becomes clear they are really seeking connection and companionship. Now, the client may find it just as helpful to join a tennis league as subscribe to a dating app.

Here's an example using a married couple. One person feels like she doesn't get enough help around the house and is beginning to get resentful. Instead of starting an argument, she puts her feelings into a positive script.

"I have been thinking a lot about all the things I have to do, and I feel overwhelmed. What I need is a partner who appreciates me and notices when they could support me more. One thing that might help is for us to tidy up the house together for fifteen minutes before we sit down to watch television. What do you think?" (Then listen for other suggestions.)

It is important to remember it is our responsibility to communicate our needs. First, find clarity as to what you really need. Needs are usually closely aligned with values. Second, be sure to communicate your needs clearly, people are not mind readers. Lastly, understand we might not get our needs met from others, but we certainly won't if we don't ask.

When identifying your needs, go deep and look underneath the feeling. If you feel fear, you probably need security or safety. If you feel anger, think of which value may have been violated. You may need respect or kindness from yourself or others. If you feel shame, what button got pushed? Do you need understanding or unconditional regard?

Brainstorm your needs. Do not get them confused with wants. You may want something but could get along fine without it. A need fulfills something deep in your soul.

Example:
Want: I want a big house.
Need: I need to live in a harmonious collaborative environment.

Come back and add to the list often.

Practice some assertive scripts.

Example One.

"I have been thinking..."

"I have been feeling... or I felt..."

"What I need is"...

"One thing that might help is..."

Example Two.

"I have been thinking..."

"I have been feeling... or I felt..."

"What I need is"...

"One thing that might help is..."

Example Three.

"I have been thinking..."

"I have been feeling... or I felt..."

"What I need is"...

"One thing that might help is..."

This script can easily be turned into an interview to gain a better understanding of another.

What have you been thinking about?

How have you been feeling lately?

What do you need from me?

Is there something I could do to help?

Modeling for others what we need is the best way to begin bringing about positive change. Try it sometime.

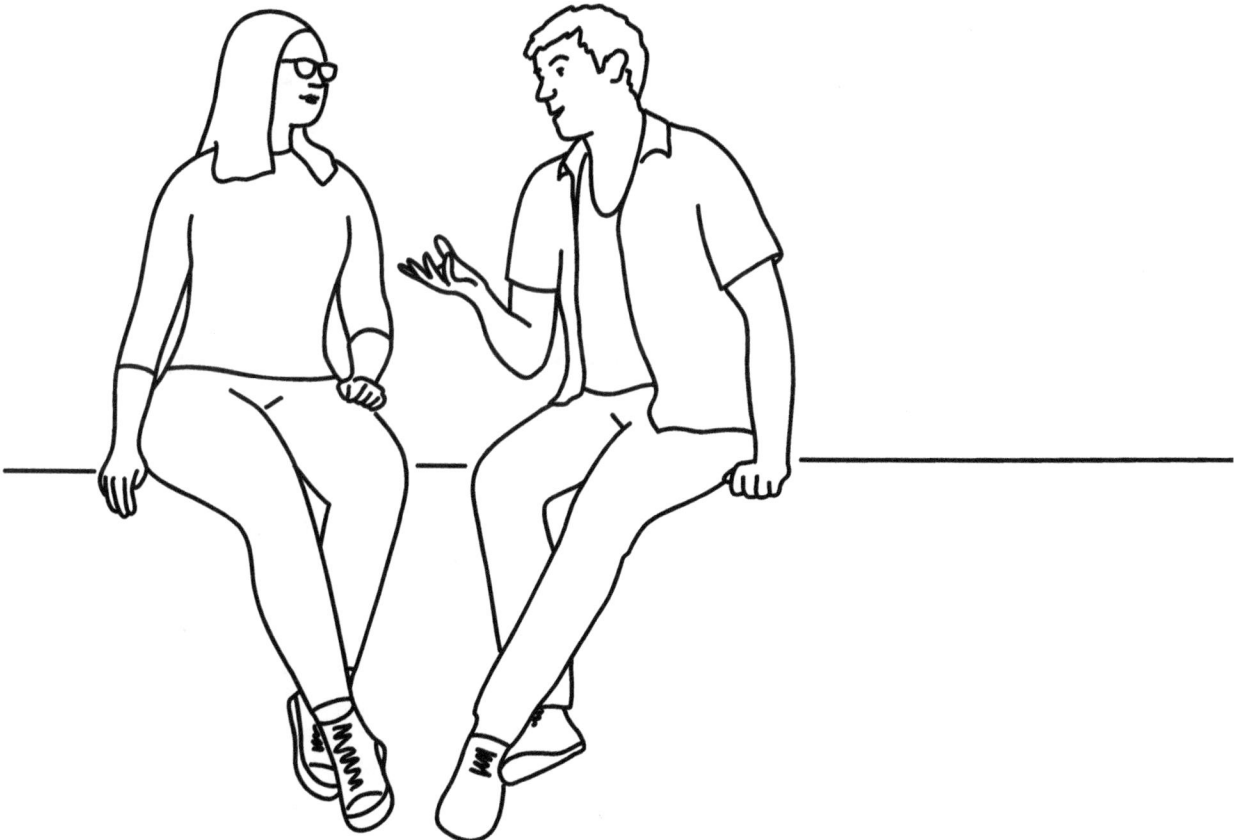

Mindful Solutions

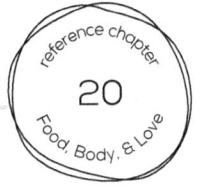

solution

Self-Compassion Meditation

May I be...*safe.*

May I be...*connected.*

May I be...*healthy.*

May I live a life...*free of fear.*

Create your own compassion meditations using your own needs and values.

May I Be... _____

May I Be... _____

May I live a life... _____

Adapted from Dr. Kristen Neff's Self-Compassion Meditations

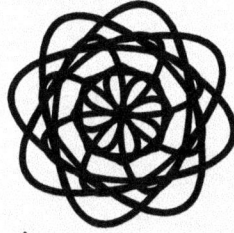

8 C's

Experience

In this session we will focus on Connection.

"Be Connected"

Draw a picture or symbol, or write a phrase, reminding you and anchoring you to the feeling of connection.

Reflect and list times when you felt connected in the past.

_____

_____

_____

_____

How can you create more connection in your life?

_____

_____

_____

Reflection and Discussion

Reflection: Use this space to write freely about any insights gained from this chapter.

_____

_____

_____

_____

_____

_____

_____

_____

_____

_____

_____

_____

_____

_____

_____

_____

_____

_____

Discussion and Activities for Group Leaders

- Ask if anyone, or all, would care to share their relationship inventory from the Moving Towards Safer Relationships activity.

- Ask if anyone, or all, would care to share about their protective habits in relationships.

- If you have a computer, share Pedigree's® "Hearts Aligned" video. Ask if anyone has a story of a special bond they share or shared with a pet. Tend to feelings.

- Ask if anyone, or all, can share an example of an experiment using "the scientist skill."

- Review the Assertive Scripts format, and ask if anyone, or all, would care to share some examples of scripts. Help to identify the difference between needs and wants.

- Practice a self-compassion meditation.

Notes

Notes

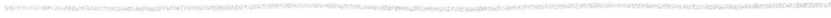

Notes

Notes

Notes

Notes

For Further Reading

Anxiety and Intrusive Thoughts

Finding Quiet: My Story of Overcoming Anxiety and the Practicing that Brought Peace
J.P. Moreland

Get Out of Your Mind and into Your Life: The New Acceptance and Commitment Therapy
Steven C. Hayes and Spencer Smith

Overcoming Unwanted Intrusive Thoughts: A CBT-Based Guide to Getting Over Frightening, Obsessive, or Disturbing Thoughts
Sally M. Winston, PsyD, and Martin N. Seif, PhD

Try Softer: A Fresh Approach to Move Us out of Anxiety, Stress and Survival Mode—and into a Life of Connection and Joy
Aundi Kolber, MA, LPC

Binge Eating

Eat What You Love, Love What You Eat for Binge Eating: A Mindful Eating Program for Healing Your Relationship with Food & Your Body
Michelle May, MD, and Kari Anderson, DBH, LPC, CEDS

Integrative Medicine for Binge Eating. A Comprehensive Guide to the New Hope Model for the Elimination of Binge Eating and Food Cravings
James Greenblatt, MD

Eating Disorders

The Eating Disorder Trap: A Guide for Clinicians and Loved Ones
Robyn L. Goldberg, REN, CEDRD-S

Nutrition

Fuel Your Brain, Not Your Anxiety: Stop the Cycle of Worry, Fatigue and Sugar Cravings with Simple Protein-Rich Foods
Kristen Allott, ND, MS, and Natasha Duarte, MS

How Not to Diet: The Groundbreaking Science of Healthy, Permanent Weight Loss
Michael Greger, MD, FACLM

The Psychobiotic Revolution: Mood, Food and the New Science of the Gut- Brain Connection
Scott Anderson, John Cryan, et al.

On Change

Atomic Habits: An Easy & Proven Way to Build Good Habits & Break Bad Ones
James Clear

The Power of Habit: Why We Do What We Do in Life and Business
Charles Duhigg

Tiny Habits. The Small Changes that Change Everything
BJ Fogg, PhD

Sleep

The Circadian Code: Lose Weight. Supercharge your Energy and Transform your Health From Morning to Midnight
Satchin Panda, PhD

Why We Sleep: Unlocking the Power of Sleep and Dreams
Matthew Walker, PhD, Steve West, et al.

Trauma Recovery

Becoming Safely Embodied: A Guide to Organize your Mind, Body and Heart to Feel Secure in the World.
Deirdre Fay, MSW, and Janina Fisher, PhD

Boundaries for Your Soul: How to Turn your Overwhelming Thoughts and Feelings into your Greatest Allies
Alison Cook, PhD, and Kimberly Miller, MTh, LMFT

Greater Than the Sum of Our Parts: Discovering Your True Self Through Internal Family Systems Therapy
Richard C. Schwartz, PhD

The Body Keeps The Score: Brain, Mind, and Body in the Healing of Trauma
Bessel Van Der Kolk, MD

What Happened to You?: Conversations on Trauma, Resilience, and Healing
Bruce D. Perry, Oprah Winfrey, et al.

Vagus Nerve and Polyvagal Theory

Accessing the Healing Power of the Vagus Nerve: Self-Help Exercises for Anxiety, Depression, Trauma, and Autism
Stanley Rosenberg, Benjamin Shield, et al.

Anchored: How to Befriend your Nervous System using Polyvagal Theory
Deborah Dana

Polyvagal Safety: Attachment, Communication, Self-Regulation
Stephen W. Porges

The Pocket Guide to the Polyvagal Theory: The Transformative Power of Feeling Safe
Stephen W. Porges

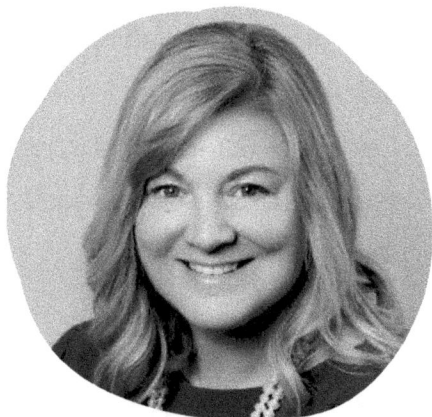

About The Author

Dr. Kari Anderson

LPC, CEDS-S.

Having personally struggled with binge eating and weight stigma, a personal passion drives Kari's professional career. Her therapeutic presence creates a safe, nonjudgmental, and healing environment making her, as patients often state, "someone who gets it."

Prior to starting her private practice, Kari positioned herself as a respected clinician and leader in the field of eating disorders. Over the course of thirty-two years, she developed several treatment models and helped thousands of patients and their families through programs such as Green Mountain at Fox Run, and Remuda Ranch.

An athlete, Kari studied physical education and nutrition in her undergraduate degree yet became interested in counseling after her own recovery from an eating disorder. In 1991, she received her counseling degree from Mount St. Mary's College in Los Angeles, California. She earned her Doctor of Behavioral Health with her research project *The Mindful Eating Cycle: Treatment for Binge Eating Disorder* at Arizona State University in 2012. Co-creator of the Am I Hungry?® Mindful Eating for Binge Eating Program, Kari also co-authored the acclaimed book, *Eat What You Love, Love What You Eat for Binge Eating: A Mindful Eating Program for Healing Your Relationship with Food & Your Body*. In 2021, she released her memoir, *Food, Body, & Love, but the greatest of these is love*. This work goes deeper into the science behind effective treatment for binge and emotional eating.

Kari holds a faculty position with Plymouth State University in New Hampshire and serves on the certification committee for the International Association of Eating Disorder Professionals, supporting supervisors for the Certified Eating Disorder Specialist (CEDS-S) designation. Kari is a licensed counselor, coach, consultant, supervisor, author, speaker, and blogger on disordered eating, behavior change strategy, and weight neutrality.

She lives in the greater Phoenix area with her husband Brian and therapy dog, Gretel. They enjoy their church community, pickleball, cycling, and vacations near the water.

You can find Kari on her website: myeatingdoctor.com. Food, Body, and Love Coaching Programs available at foodbodyandlove.com

Join the foodbodyandlove support community on Facebook https://www.facebook.com/groups/308901044114453

Food, Body and Love Online Course and Communityt at https://drkaricourses.thinkific.com/courses/food-body-and-love

Kari is available for training licensed professionals, lay counselors and coaches to facilitate the Food, Body, & Love program.